A Woman's Ayurvedic Herbal

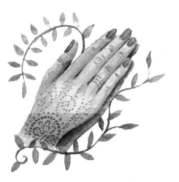

D1736685

A Guide for Natural Health and Well-Being

CAROLINE ROBERTSON & ANTONIA BEATTIE

HAMPTON ROADS

Designer: Stephanie Doyle
Illustrator: Jeff Lang/Tina Wilson
Typeset in Giovanni and Georgia

Hampton Roads Publishing Company, Inc.
Charlottesville, VA 22906
Distributed by Red Wheel/Weiser, LLC
www.redwheelweiser.com

Sign up for our newsletter and special offers by going to
www.redwheelweiser.com/newsletter.

ISBN: 978-1-64297-012-8
Library of Congress Cataloging-in-Publication Data
available upon request.

Printed in Korea
TWP
10 9 8 7 6 5 4 3 2 1

DISCLAIMER

This book is intended to give general information only and is not a substitute for professional and medical advice. Consult your health-care provider before adopting any of the treatments contained in this book. The publisher, author, and distributor expressly disclaim all liability to any person arising directly or indirectly from the use of, or for any errors or omissions in, the information in this book. The adoption and application of the information in this book is at the reader's discretion and is their sole responsibility.

  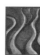 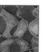 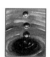

Contents

Healing through Ayurveda

A–Z of Common Ailments

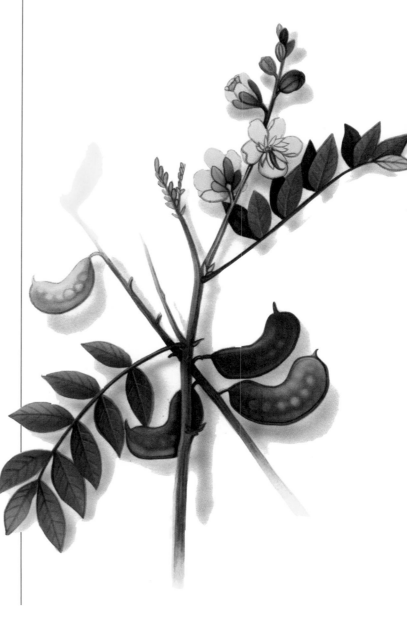

Introduction
Healing using Ayurvedic principles

What is Ayurveda? Known as "the mother of all healing sciences," it is the oldest holistic health system. Developed in India an estimated 4,000 years ago, Ayurveda is a complete system for healing and rebalancing the body. Ayurveda focuses on empowering individuals to heal rapidly and easily with the aid of herbs, diet, body therapies and lifestyle tools. Ayurveda uses a range of specific herbs and spices, some very well known in the West, such as cinnamon, cumin, turmeric and pepper, to detoxify the body and to calm or stimulate the metabolism. Indian traditional herbs such as brahmi (the brain-boosting herb) are becoming very popular in the West as scientific research confirms their potency.

The term Ayurveda is derived from two Sanskrit words that, combined, mean the wisdom or science of life. The Ayurvedic system of healing is holistic in that all aspects of a person's life and emotions are factored into the healing process. The right food, sleep patterns, exercise, relationships and spirituality are all considered important to the health of a person. To determine what is right for an individual, Ayurvedic practitioners abide by the principle that there are three primary body types—*vata*, *pitta* and *kapha* (see pages 8–10). Each body type or constitution (*prakriti*) is predisposed to particular imbalances and is responsive to specific healing techniques and lifestyle regimes.

Ayurvedic wisdom is strongly based on the fundamental belief that the elements that make up the world—ether, air, fire, water and earth—are also present in the makeup of the human body. Every body has a predominance of a particular combination of elements (see page 8). Ayurveda is an especially effective form of healing because it is based on an understanding of the interrelationship between human beings and nature, and works to promote harmony between the two. True health and balance is experienced when all these elements are in balance. When they are out of balance, symptoms of disease can arise.

Ayurvedic medicine is also based on analyzing a person's body type (see pages 8–11), then treating an ailment according to the requirements of that type. An Ayurvedic practitioner may also suggest a diet that balances a person's constitution; a detoxification process; lifestyle changes; massage and the use of color, aromas, oils, crystals, or medicinal herbs and spices. The most common herbs and spices now easily available in the West are described and discussed on pages 16–69 in terms of their:

• historical or mythological background;
• use in Ayurvedic medicine;
• home remedies; and
• available forms.

Ayurvedic practitioners consider that one of the most important functions of the human body is digestion. Often, the early symptoms of disease can be alleviated by balancing the digestive fire or *agni*. The lack of digestive juices or "fire" leads to the accumulation of undigested material, or *ama*, in the body. This material is toxic waste that circulates through the body creating symptoms that reduce the quality of life and one's life span. By balancing the digestive fire, these waste products dissolve and are easily expelled by the body. Spices are incorporated into Ayurvedic medicine to maintain a proper level of digestive fire that will promote good health, a sense of vitality, and a long life. Each ailment listed in this book (pages 100–155) is discussed in terms of both its symptoms and the recommended treatments to alleviate the symptoms, bringing the body back into balance by the use of medicinal herbs and spices and by making simple changes to your lifestyle. A case study will also be given to illustrate practical management of each ailment.

You can use this list of ailments to discover how Ayurveda can help you to cope with specific problems that you may be experiencing. However, since prevention is always better than cure, also take time to look at Ayurveda's advice on averting disease by matching a person's body type with the most beneficial lifestyle. Read pages 72–97 to learn how, by adopting a routine and lifestyle suited to your body type, you can live a healthy, happy and fulfilling life. The Ayurvedic approach to health is an exciting one that, if pursued in a mindful manner, can provide a sense of harmony in not only the body but also the mind and spirit, initiating a heightened sense of stability and serenity.

THE EIGHT BRANCHES OF AYURVEDA

1. General Medicine (Kaya Chikitsa)
2. Pediatrics (Bala Chikitsa)
3. Psychology and Psychiatry (Graha Chikitsa)
4. Ear, Nose and Throat and Ophthalmology (Shalakya Chikitsa)
5. Surgery (Shalya Chikitsa)
6. Toxicology (Visha Chikitsa)
7. Rejuvenation/Geriatrics (Rasayana Chikitsa)
8. Infertility (Vajikarana Chikitsa)

Chikitsa is a Sanskrit word meaning treatment or therapy.

The three doshas & body types:

Which body type are you?

In Ayurvedic medicine, there are three major principles, namely vata, pitta and kapha, around which the entire science revolves. Vata is the active principle from ether and air, pitta from fire and water, and kapha from water and earth.

Dosha   Functions

Vata   enthusiasm, mobility, circulation, regulation

Pitta   heat, transformation, analysis, effulgence, courage

Kapha   integrity, lubrication, stability, patience, calmness

Everything in this universe is composed of all the five elements, but in varying proportions. Each of us has a unique proportion of these *doshas*, known as prakriti or body types. Understanding our proportion of these elements or doshas is vital in designing and deciding what is good and what is bad for us.

To get a specific idea of your prakriti, complete the questionnaire on pages 9–11. The following summary provides a broad idea of body type characteristics.

- a vata type is naturally slim with narrow hips and shoulders and a fluctuating flow of energy;
- a pitta type is generally medium height, size and weight with an even flow of energy; and
- a kapha type is usually thickset with wide shoulders and hips and a tendency to be slow and steady.

The following questions will help you to determine your body type. Understanding your prakriti is the first step toward a happy life and effective health care. This wisdom guides us to understand the most suitable daily routine, nutrition, colors, essential oils, herbs and other therapeutic substances for ourselves. Count all the checks in each section and grade your answers as either rarely or mostly. Your predominant dosha is the one in which the score is higher than the others. If the scores for two doshas are nearly identical, then you have a combination prakriti.

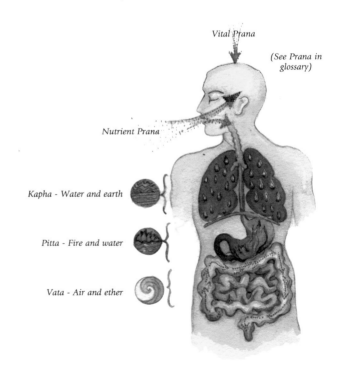

Vital Prana

(See Prana in glossary)

Nutrient Prana

Kapha - Water and earth

Pitta - Fire and water

Vata - Air and ether

CHECKLIST FOR AYURVEDIC BODY TYPES

VATA TYPE
AIR AND ETHER DOMINANT

	Rarely	Mostly
I am hyperactive or do things rapidly	☐	☐
I learn and forget easily	☐	☐
I am enthusiastic and vivacious	☐	☐
I have a thin physique	☐	☐
I walk quickly and lightly	☐	☐
I can be indecisive	☐	☐
I have a tendency to constipation	☐	☐
I often have cold feet and hands	☐	☐
I am frequently anxious and nervous	☐	☐
I am talkative and speak quickly	☐	☐
I am sensitive to the cold	☐	☐
My mood often changes quickly	☐	☐
My sleep is light and short	☐	☐
My skin is dry, especially in the winter	☐	☐
I have an active, restless and imaginative mind	☐	☐
My energy tends to come in bursts	☐	☐
I use up my energy quickly	☐	☐
My eating and sleeping habits tend to be irregular	☐	☐
I don't gain weight easily, but do lose it easily	☐	☐
My appetite is variable	☐	☐
In my dreams I fly, jump or travel, and I'm often fearful	☐	☐
My faith is changeable or wavering	☐	☐
I often feel insecure, fearful or anxious	☐	☐
I sometimes develop painful or nervous conditions	☐	☐
My teeth have spaces between them or are irregular	☐	☐
TOTAL	___	___

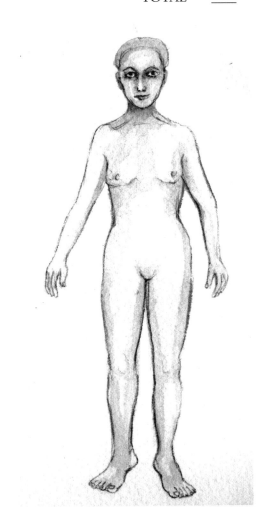

9

PITTA TYPE
FIRE AND WATER DOMINANT

	Rarely	Mostly
I am usually efficient	☐	☐
I tend to be extremely precise and orderly	☐	☐
I am strong-minded and have a forceful manner	☐	☐
I feel uncomfortable or easily tired in hot weather	☐	☐
I perspire easily	☐	☐
Even though I might not always show it, I become irritable quite easily	☐	☐
If I skip a meal or a meal is delayed, I become uncomfortable	☐	☐
One or more of the following characteristics describe my hair —early graying, balding or reddish	☐	☐
I have a strong appetite	☐	☐
I have regular bowel habits— it would be more common for me to have diarrhea than constipation	☐	☐
I like to set goals for myself and then try to achieve them	☐	☐
I become impatient very easily	☐	☐
I tend to be a perfectionist about details	☐	☐
I get angry quite easily, but then quickly forget about it	☐	☐
I am very fond of cold foods and drinks	☐	☐
I am more likely to feel that a room is too hot than too cold	☐	☐
I don't tolerate foods that are very hot and spicy	☐	☐
I am not as tolerant of disagreement as I should be	☐	☐
I enjoy challenges. When I want something, I am very determined and strive to attain it	☐	☐
I tend to be quite critical of myself and others	☐	☐
My dreams are usually colorful and passionate	☐	☐
I have a determined faith	☐	☐
I tend to be aggressive	☐	☐
My illnesses are often related to infection or inflammation	☐	☐
I have soft bleeding gums and teeth that are moderate in size	☐	☐
TOTAL	_____	_____

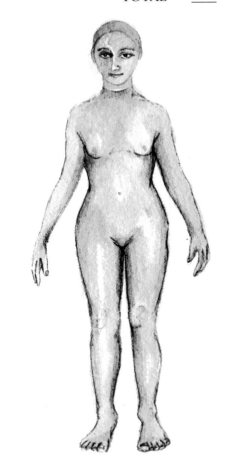

KAPHA TYPE
EARTH AND WATER DOMINANT

	Rarely	Mostly
I do things in a slow and relaxed but steady fashion	☐	☐
I gain weight easily and lose it slowly	☐	☐
I am quiet by nature and usually only talk when necessary	☐	☐
I can skip meals easily without much discomfort	☐	☐
I have a tendency toward excess mucus, phlegm, congestion, asthma or sinus problems	☐	☐
I must get at least eight hours of sleep in order to feel comfortable the next day	☐	☐
I sleep very deeply	☐	☐
I am not easily angered— I am generally calm by nature	☐	☐
I don't learn as quickly as some people, but I have better retention and a good long-term memory	☐	☐
I eat slowly	☐	☐
Cool or damp weather sometimes bothers me	☐	☐
My hair is thick and strong	☐	☐
I have smooth, soft skin or a pale complexion	☐	☐
I have a large, solid body build	☐	☐
I often feel unmotivated	☐	☐
I have slow digestion	☐	☐
I have very good stamina and physical endurance	☐	☐
I generally walk with a slow, measured gait	☐	☐
I am slow to get going in the morning	☐	☐

I usually do things slowly and methodically	☐	☐
My dreams are watery, emotional, romantic or I'm swimming	☐	☐
My faith is steady and loyal	☐	☐
I am attached, self-centered and occasionally greedy	☐	☐
I am usually prone to diseases such as fluid retention or mucus buildup	☐	☐
My teeth are strong, white, well-formed and full	☐	☐
TOTAL	___	___

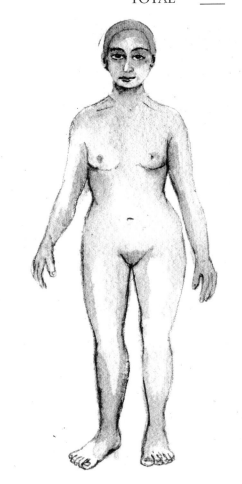

The use of herbs in Ayurvedic medicine

In Ayurveda, herbs are classified according to their effect on the human body. An herb's impact is seen in a number of different ways, including its taste, whether it has a heating or cooling effect, and its impact on a person's digestion. In Ayurvedic medicine, herbs, as well as food and drink, are used in regard to their tastes. Ayurveda identifies six major tastes—sweet, sour, salty, pungent, bitter, and astringent.

Sweet-tasting herbs, such as fennel, licorice and marshmallow, may be used for the connective tissue, as well as for healing broken bones and helping loosen phlegm during a cold by acting as an expectorant. Salty and sour tastes are excellent for aiding digestion, while astringent tastes, such as tumeric and pomegranate, are good for wound healing and blood clearing. Pungent-tasting herbs include a large number of spices used for culinary purposes, such as asafetida, black and long peppers, cardamom, cinnamon, cloves, coriander, cumin, garlic and ginger. These are used to stimulate circulation and promote digestion. Bitter herbs, such as aloe vera, help relieve nausea, stimulate the digestive juices, and aid in the elimination of toxins, including worms.

Herbs are also classified according to whether they have a heating or cooling effect. This classification relates to their taste. Pungent, sour, and salty-tasting herbs have a heating energy. Heating the body is very useful, particularly for aiding the digestive system. Ayurvedic medicine teaches that all disease arises from poor digestion or insufficient "fire." This fire is called *agni*. Agni is evident in all living things and is the driving force behind life processes. Agni corresponds with the state of our metabolism, which is in turn governed by the state of our digestion.

If digestion is poor, toxins can be broken down and *ama* is reduced once the digestive fire is stabilized. Ama is the toxin created by undigested food. An excess of ama in the body leads to lethargy, digestive disorders, and cloudy thinking. In Ayurvedsic medicine, balance is the key to health. It is important to raise only as much agni as is needed to burn off the ama. Too much agni will result in acidic conditions, such as heartburn.

As heating herbs have the ability to increase agni, cooling herbs can help increase *soma*. Soma corresponds with the element of water and governs the nerves and mind. Cooling herbs are usually sweet, astringent, or bitter. However, some herbs can be both, such as Indian Gooseberry, which is predominantly sour with a cooling energy, indicating that they can be useful for certain inflammatory disorders. s

AID YOUR DIGESTION BY CHOOSING HERBS ACCORDING TO YOUR BODY TYPE	
Type	*Herbs to increase* agni
Kapha	Aloe vera, black pepper, cardamom, cinnamon, cumin, fennel, garlic, ginger
Pitta	Aloe vera, coriander, cumin, fennel
Vata	Asafetida, black pepper, cardamom, cinnamon, cumin, fennel, garlic, ginger

Your body type is relevant to what heating or cooling herbs to take for any health problems, because these three body types suffer from different imbalances. For this reason, heating herbs are excellent for kapha and vata types, but may aggravate pitta body types. When out of balance, a kapha type tends toward mucus accumulation, lethargy, weight gain and diabetes. Weight loss, gas and loss of strength are some of the indications that vata imbalance exists. As the kapha metabolism has a "cold and heavy energy" and vata has a "cold and light energy," improving agni will help these two body types rebalance themselves. Health imbalances experienced by pitta body types may include inflammation and infection. Pitta body types benefit the most from cooling herbs, as this body type has a "fiery" energy. Also, a number of herbs are *tridoshic*, which means that they are suitable for all body types or doshas. Such herbs include aloe vera, coriander, cumin, fennel, rose flowers, saffron and gotu kola.

Herbs are prepared in a great variety of ways in Ayurvedic medicine. Herbs such as aloe vera are particularly potent when taken as a fresh juice (*svarasa*). Preparing herbs with hot water is called either a decoction (*kashaya*) or a hot infusion (*phanta*) and is prepared by heating the herbs and the water together. This technique can be used to make pills (*gulika*) and tablets (*vati*). A hot infusion (*phanta*) is one in which hot water is poured over the herbs and the herbs are left to steep for a short time. Leaving the herbs to stand in cold water is called a cold infusion (*sheeta kashaya*).

Ayurvedic herbal powders (*churnas*) are often combinations of 5 to 20 or more herbs ground into a fine powder that can be mixed with substances to aid their assimilation, such as ghee or honey. Ghee is clarified butter, and can increase agni for all body types. It is used for both cooking and for medicinal purposes. Medicated ghee (*gritha*) is prepared with herbs appropriate for both pitta and vata body types. Kapha types are advised to limit their use of ghee as it can promote weight gain. Other herbal combinations include medicated jellies (*avaleha*) and medicated wines (*asavas* and *arishtas*). Thousands of ancient, traditional combinations of herbs are still prescribed by Ayurvedic practitioners, such as *trikatu* (a compound of ginger, black and long pepper), which is excellent for purifying the body and to ignite agni.

The form of the herb most effective for a condition depends largely on the adjunct it is given with. These adjuncts are called *anupanas* and enhance the absorption and efficacy of the herbs.

TIPS ON PREPARING HERBS	
Imbalance in:	*Substance taken with the herb:*
Vata	Oil
Pitta	Ghee
Kapha	Honey

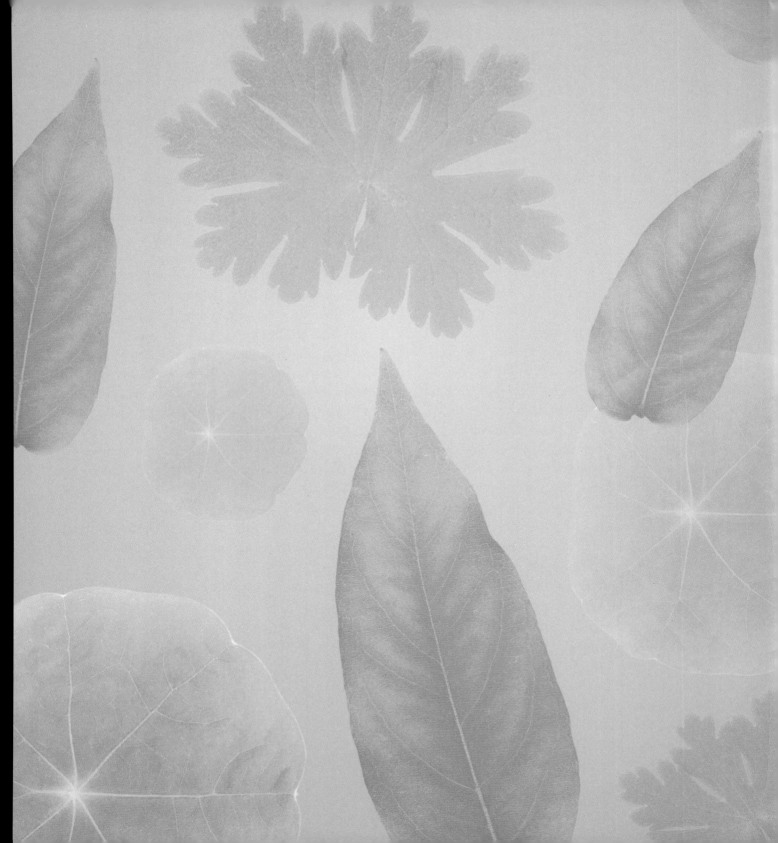

A-Z of Herbs and Spices

Aloe Vera

Aloe barbadensis, Indian aloe, the "first aid plant"
Sanskrit: Kumari *Hindi:* Kumari, Gawarpaltra
FAMILY: Liliaceae

Believed to be a gift from the goddess Venus, aloe vera has been used as a cure-all for conditions ranging from the healing of wounds to the proper digestion of food.

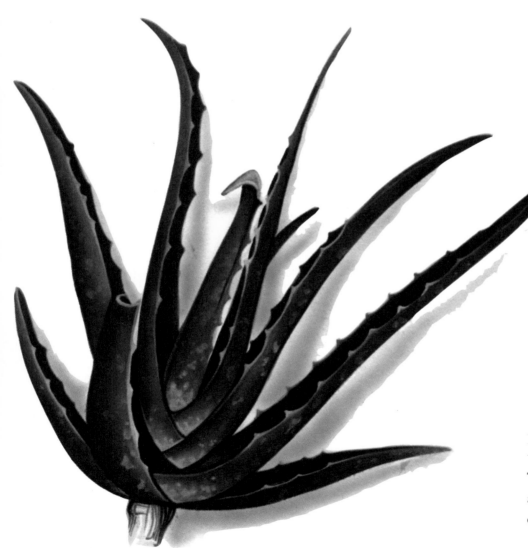

Description

A perennial, succulent plant that grows low to the ground with narrow, tapering, thorn-edged, fleshy leaves that contain a gelatinous juice. The color of the leaves varies from gray to dark green, with some varieties featuring light green leaves with horizontal markings. Leaves grow to between 1–2 feet (30–60 cm) long and are arranged in a circular fashion around a fibrous root. The plant produces tube-shaped flowers that are yellow, red or purple. The plant grows easily in most areas of India and other parts of the world.

Historical or mythological background

Known as the "Plant of Immortality" by the ancient Egyptians and the "Universal Panacea" by the ancient Greeks, the aloe vera plant has been used internally as a digestive aid and externally for burns as well as a soothing lotion for the skin. The Sanskrit name "Kumari" means "virgin girl," which alludes to the regenerative power of aloe vera with respect to the female reproductive system. Its ability to survive in tropical and difficult conditions with little water has led to metaphysical connotations of aloe bringing success in the face of adversity.

Modern uses

If taken internally, aloe juice cleanses the blood, liver and reproductive system. This cleansing action is particularly effective for relieving pitta conditions such as rashes, acne, liver disorders, menopausal flashes and painful periods. Externally, aloe vera is also effective for vaginal herpes, burns, actinic keratoses/keratoacanthomas (sunspots), fungal infections and eczema. Applied to the nails, it acts as an effective nail-biting deterrent.

Available forms

Aloe juice is widely available from health food stores. Avoid juices preserved with ascorbic or citric acid as they are heating, and thus counter aloe's cooling effect. Gel and cream for external use can be obtained easily, but avoid those with lanolin, as it is also heating. Capsules of concentrated powder are also sold at health food stores. Follow the recommended dose, as excessive quantities may cause cramps and diarrhea. An aloe-based Ayurvedic wine—called *Kumaryasavan*—is used for female reproductive imbalances and liver conditions.

Home remedies

For wounds, apply $\frac{1}{2}$ tsp aloe gel with $\frac{1}{2}$ tsp comfrey cream, $\frac{1}{5}$ tsp ghee and $\frac{1}{5}$ tsp turmeric. For sensitive or deep burns, fill an atomizer with:

- 50 ml warm water, 2 tsp pure aloe vera gel and $\frac{1}{3}$ tsp turmeric;
- Shake well, then add 1 tsp pure honey;
- Cool in fridge before spraying on the affected area twice daily.

If you suffer from inflamed eyelids, apply a mixture of $\frac{1}{2}$ tsp aloe gel and $\frac{1}{5}$ tsp rose water.

Caution: externally, aloe vera juice can cause allergic dermatitis in those with very sensitive skin.

> *Kumari expels toxins, and is a cold, bitter, sweet tonic with nourishing and rejuvenative properties. It strengthens vision, enhances fertility, eliminates poisons and balances vata.*
> —Bhava Prakasha Samhita *[An ancient Ayurvedic text]*

Asafetida (also known as Hing)

Ferula asafetida, Hing, "Devil's dung," "Food of the Gods'
Sanskrit: Hingu *Hindi:* Hing
FAMILY: Umbelliferae

Used in Indian cooking over 2,500 years ago, asafetida is renowned for its ability to alleviate nervous disorders and gastric irritation when used in small doses.

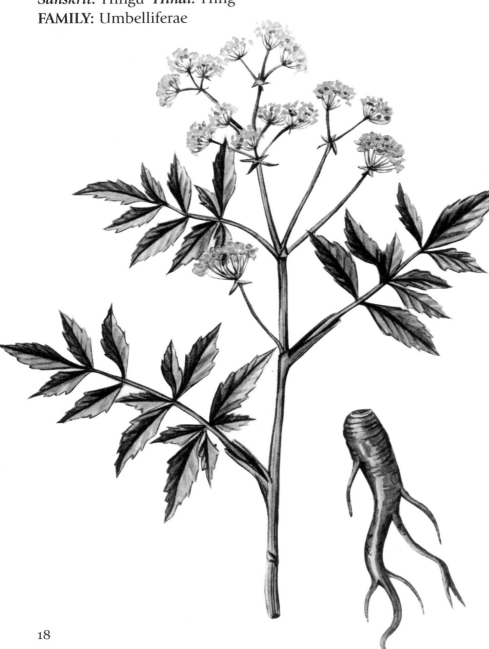

Description

A perennial plant with a large, fleshy root covered with coarse fibers, from which grows a central thick stem with many small branches. The dense branches sport pale yellow flowers, and the plant bears fruit of a reddish-brown color. The stem, which is covered with a black bark, is cut just before flowering. The cut exudes a thick, milky, pungent-smelling resin that is collected when the sap has hardened, then dried and powdered. Only a mature plant, one that has grown to between 5–9 ft (1.8–3 m) high, is cut. Asafetida grows best in stony, dry soil in high altitudes, such as are found in Afghanistan, Kashmir, Iran, Tibet and the Punjab.

Historical or mythological background

Believed to have first grown from the semen of a god of fertility, the herb has long been associated with increasing sexual libido. Asafetida has been used in Indian cooking since ancient times and has also been planted in gardens as an insect deterrent. Because asafetida contains a volatile oil containing sulphur, the powder has also been used in magical ceremonies to banish negative energies in the shape of demons and other evil spirits.

Modern uses

Asafetida is one of Ayurveda's primary remedies to combat excess vata. It breaks down toxins and promotes their elimination through its diuretic and laxative action. The powdered resin is a powerful remedy for flatulent colic, asthma, painful periods and arthritis. For centuries, it has been used in mild cases of epilepsy, hysteria and a range of psychological imbalances. A pinch of asafetida added to beans and potatoes neutralizes their gassy effect. The lightly roasted powder, combined with warm sesame oil, can be gently massaged into a baby's stomach to rapidly relieve colic.

Available forms

The most powerful form of asafetida is the pure resin sold in Indian and Asian grocery stores. This needs to be grated or boiled for use. The second best option is the powder, which is often sold in regular supermarkets and Asian stores. This is sometimes mixed with wheat and turmeric, and is therefore unsuitable for those with a wheat sensitivity.

Home remedies

For gas, abdominal distension, period pain and poor appetite, mix 1 tsp each powdered ginger, cumin, black cumin,

> *Asafetida is tasty, pungent and hot; expels worms and cures vata and kapha disorders, especially bloating, intestinal obstruction and pain. It also improves eyesight.*
> —Raja Nighantu
> *[An ancient Ayurvedic text]*

long pepper, asafetida, ajwan and rock salt. Take $3/4$ tsp of this mixture in $1/5$ cup warm water or buttermilk after meals three times a day. To relieve infant colic, roast $1/3$ tsp asafetida powder in 2 tbsp sesame oil. Allow the mixture to cool slightly and massage it on the baby's stomach in the direction of the colon (clockwise when facing the baby).

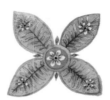

Basil (Holy)

Ocimum sanctum, Sacred basil
Sanskrit: Tulasi *Hindi:* Tulsi
FAMILY: Latiatae

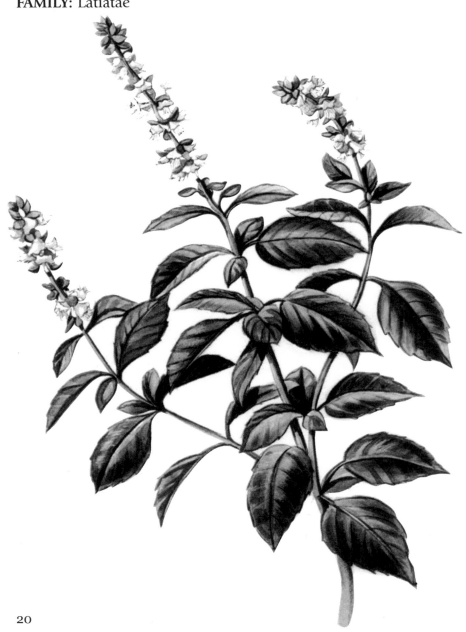

Along with the lotus, basil is one India's most sacred herbs. It is used for soothing the nerves, clearing the sinuses and strengthening feelings of compassion and courage.

Description

Holy Basil is an annual bush that grows to a height of 1–2 ft (30–60 cm). The plant features small to medium aromatic grayish-green leaves, and its flowers are lavender in color. There are two kinds of Holy Basil. One, called Sri tulsi, is the most common and is grayish-green in color; the second kind is called Krishna tulsi and is characterized by its purple leaves. The plant is grown throughout India and Europe and requires well-drained soil and a sunny and well-sheltered position.

Historical or mythological background

Holy basil is grown around Indian temples and in Hindu households. Used as a symbol of hospitality, it repels insects if hung from doorframes and windowsills. Tulasi, the Sanskrit word for "Holy Basil," or "the incomparable one," was Krishna's beautiful consort until she was cursed to take birth in the form of a tree. Worshipping this sacred tree and wearing neck beads made from its wood is said to bestow spiritual blessings upon the wearer.

Modern uses

Ayurvedic sages claim that by planting a holy basil tree in one's yard and consuming five leaves daily, illness is kept at bay. This herb is especially therapeutic for those with asthma, bronchitis, sinusitis, throat ailments or a sensitive respiratory system. Holy basil is also a potent blood purifier, useful for many infectious conditions, including stings, toxemia from poisonous bites and mercury poisoning from amalgam fillings. Gentle and safe, it is ideal for children at the onset of fevers, earaches, sore throats and stomachaches. Applied topically, the leaf juice is very soothing for bites, stings, boils, acne and ringworm.

Available forms

Though common basil is readily available, holy basil is generally sold only by Ayurvedic clinics or Indian grocery stores. The unadulterated leaves and buds can be made into a tea or crushed into juice. To enjoy holy basil's full advantages, grow one in the northeast area of your garden.

Home remedies

In Gandhi's ashram, holy basil tea was served with ginger. This is an appealing substitute for those wanting to give up caffeinated tea. Miraculous results can be achieved in relieving acne, tinea, bites, stings and ringworm if pure holy basil juice is smeared over the affected area. Place the leaves in a juice blender with a little pure water to make a juice. For coughs, colds and sinus problems, try the following recipe: in a mortar and pestle, grind 10 holy basil leaves with 3 black peppercorns. Place this in 2 cups boiling water, add 1 tsp grated ginger, and simmer uncovered until reduced by half. Strain, allowing the mixture to cool for a few minutes before stirring in 1 tsp honey. Take one cup of this tea three to four times a day.

Holy basil is pungent, bitter, hot and fragrant; balances kapha and vata; cures worms, microbial infections and anorexia.
—Raja Nighantu
[An ancient Ayurvedic text]

Brahmi (also known as *Bacopa Monnieri*)

Bacopa monnieri, Thyme-leaved gratiola,
Water hyssop, Indian pennywort
Sanskrit: Brahmi, Sarasvati *Hindi:* Barama-manduki
FAMILY: Scrophulariaceae

With a name meaning divine creative energy, Brahmi is used to stimulate the brain and improve a person's memory and ability to learn. It helps relieve stress, and is also an excellent hair tonic.

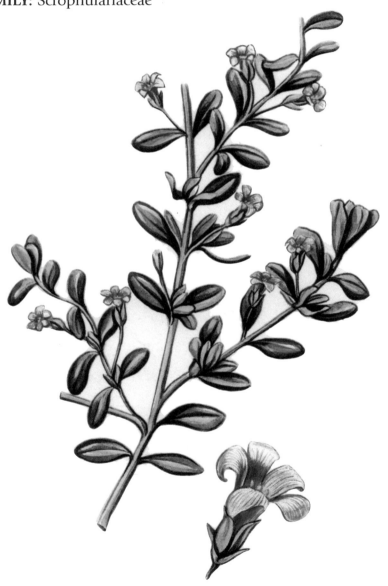

Description

Brahmi is a creeping plant that spreads on the ground in marshy areas, forming into mats. The herb has dark-green succulent leaves that are rounded, relatively thick, and spatulate or wedge-shaped. The leaves are connected to the stem by light-green succulent branches. Its flowers are small and either blue or whitish in color. Brahmi grows in the Himalayas near fresh or brackish water or marshy areas.

Historical or mythological background

The herb's connection with learning and clarity of purpose is well established. Its Sanskrit name, "Saraswati," refers to the goddess Saraswati, the epitome of Supreme Wisdom and Learning. In Hinduism, Lord Brahma is the creator of the universe. Since the plant helps the mind to focus, yogis and meditators take brahmi to enhance their spiritual focus.

Modern uses

Brahmi is Ayurveda's top brain rejuvenator. Recent research has established its efficacy in restoring memory, improving concentration and repairing the brain's neural pathways. As such, brahmi is an invaluable herb for brain injuries, Alzheimer's disease, strokes, nervous breakdowns, epilepsy and mental fatigue. Whereas many mental stimulants produce hyperactivity, brahmi is relaxing. It also increases one's resilience to stress and trauma. Brahmi hair oil has been used for millennia as an effective remedy for insomnia, psoriasis, fever and hair loss. Though not its primary use, brahmi is also combined with other herbs to help relieve rheumatism and asthma.

Available forms

Many traditional Ayurvedic brahmi preparations are in a ghee medium, which helps it to cross the brain–blood barrier. One of these preparations is called Brahmi ghritham. Brahmi tablets or fluid extracts are available from health food stores, the internet and through direct marketing companies. Pure brahmi powder is sold at Ayurvedic clinics.

Home remedies

To improve your concentration and to prevent gray hair, you can make a simplified version of the traditional oil—Brahmi thailam—at home by heating 200 ml sesame oil with 100 ml coconut oil, and adding to it ½ cup fresh whole brahmi plant, 1 tbsp ground fresh gooseberries, 1 tbsp licorice root and a 25 gram (1 oz) piece of sandalwood (this can be replaced by 10 drops of pure sandalwood essential oil, which can be added at the end). Bring everything to a boil, then simmer for 20–30 minutes. Strain and cool before storing in a dark glass bottle. Apply this slightly warmed oil to the scalp, leaving on for 30 minutes daily.

Caution: If you have high blood pressure, only take brahmi under medical supervision.

> *Brahmi is bitter in taste, pungent in post digestion and lubricating. It is life enhancing, cures respiratory conditions, kapha and mental imbalances. Brahmi slows ageing, improving the memory, voice and metabolism.*
> —*Sodhala Nighantu*
> *[An ancient Ayurvedic text]*

Cardamom

Elettaria cardamomum, Cardamom seeds
Sanskrit: Ela *Hindi:* Elachi
FAMILY: Ginger

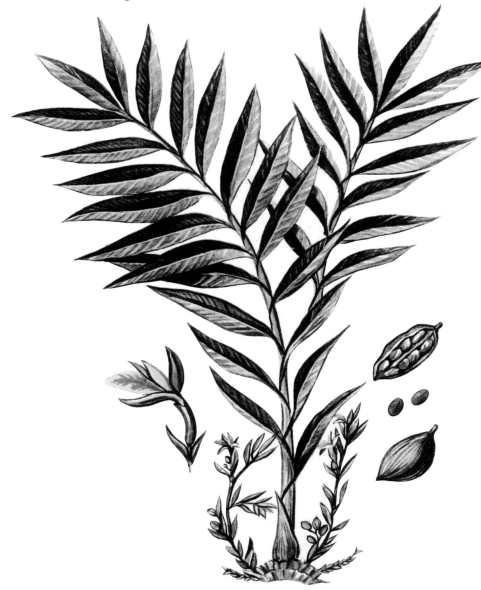

An excellent digestive aid, cardamom is useful for asthma and other respiratory conditions, as well as helping the mind and heart to experience joy and clarity.

Description

Cardamom is a perennial plant that grows as an upright stem supporting leaves and flowers or fruit. The narrow, tapering leaves are two-toned, being dark green, with a smooth texture on the upper side and light green underneath. The flowers are small and yellow, and the plant has an oval-shaped fruit pod containing the seeds of the cardamom. The plant is grown successfully in southern India and in other areas of India, as well as in Guatemala, Tanzania, Sri Lanka and Burma. It is best grown in soil that is loamy (a rich, dark soil), and in a warm, humid climate.

Historical or mythological background

In Ayurvedic medicine, cardamom has been used since the 4th century BC, especially as a digestive and as an aid to alleviate the symptoms of obesity. There are two types of Indian cardamom—Malabar cardamom and Mysore cardamom. In India, cardamom was also renowned for its ability to give clarity and a sense of joy to the user. Ancient Arabs used the herb as an aphrodisiac, and the Greeks and Romans used cardamom as a perfume. The ancient Egyptians chewed the seeds to help keep their teeth clean.

Modern uses

As cardamom bestows a sweet voice and breath, the seeds are often added to desserts or chewed after a meal. Those with a vata or kapha imbalance find the spice particularly beneficial for coughs, colds and asthma, as it clears the passages of mucus congestion.

Cardamom also reduces the gassy indigestion to which vata types are prone. For loss of appetite and indigestion, cardamom seeds are often given with ginger. Recent research indicates that cardamom has the unique action of detoxifying the body of caffeine and codeine.

Available forms

Cardamom pods, powder or seeds are readily available from supermarkets, green-grocers and spice shops. The pods are best when a little green and can be gently crushed before use as an infusion or as an addition to rice or vegetable dishes. The seeds are more potent when freshly crushed in a mortar and pestle or spice grinder.

> *Cardamom is pungent, cold, light and balances vata and kapha. It is excellent for treating respiratory and kidney conditions.*
> —Bhava Prakasha Samhita
> *[An ancient Ayurvedic text]*

Since the resulting powder is very concentrated, only small quantities are required, about $1/5$ tsp per person, depending on the dish.

Home remedies

An excellent combination with cardamom for mucous flus, colds, coughs and indigestion is called *Thaalesapathraadi churnam*.

For a homemade version, mix together:

- 2 tsp black pepper powder;
- 3 tsp ginger powder;
- $3\frac{1}{2}$ tsp long pepper powder;
- $\frac{1}{2}$ tsp cardamom powder;
- $\frac{1}{2}$ tsp cinnamon powder; and
- $\frac{1}{2}$ tsp ground palm sugar.

Take $\frac{1}{2}$ tsp mixed powder with 1 tsp honey in $\frac{1}{4}$ cup warm water three to four times daily until the symptoms subside.

Add a pinch of cardamom and black pepper to yogurt, cheese or warm milk to reduce the mucus buildup that may result from eating or drinking dairy products.

Cinnamon

Cinnamomum cassia, "Blume', Ceylon cinnamon, True cinnamon
Sanskrit: Tvak **Hindi:** Dalchini, Darucini
FAMILY: Lauraceae

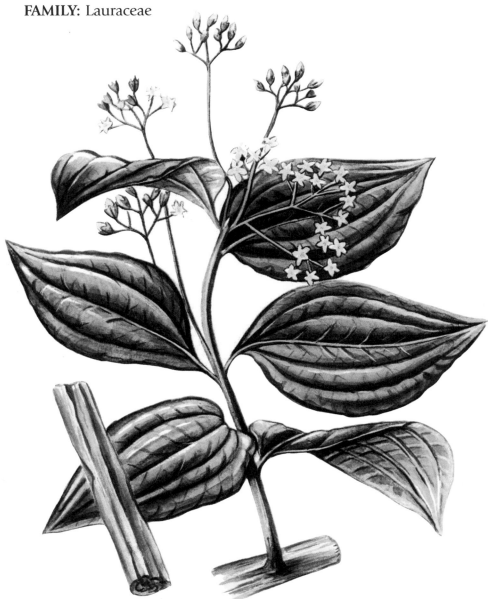

*A **sweet, aromatic spice, cinnamon is used for both culinary and medicinal purposes. It stimulates digestion and energizes the circulation, heart and kidneys.***

Description

True cinnamon is the dried inner bark of the laurel tree, while common cinnamon is often from the cassia tree. The laurel tree is a tropical evergreen that grows up to 56 ft (17 m) high. It has ovate leaves that are two-toned—dark green on top and light green underneath. The tree has small white or yellow flowers that bear purple berries. The bark is smooth and yellowish in color, and is rolled, pressed and dried to make cinnamon sticks. If from the cassia tree, the sticks or quills are light brown to tan in color; the sticks from the laurel tree are much lighter in color and finer in quality. Cinnamon is native to Sri Lanka and southern India.

Historical or mythological background

Cinnamon has been used as a medicine since ancient times. The Egyptians imported cinnamon in huge quantities for a variety of reasons, including the flavoring of beverages and for their embalming processes, as cinnamon also acts as a preservative. In Roman times, the Emperor Nero burned a huge supply of cinnamon at his wife's funeral to signify his deep sense of loss at her death. In the 15th and 16th centuries, the spice inspired a number of explorations and, after the invasion of Sri Lanka by Portugal, the King of Sri Lanka was forced to give a large amount of cinnamon as a tribute to the Portuguese.

Modern uses

The wonderful warming quality of cinnamon stimulates the circulation and heats chilled lungs and kidneys. Cinnamon essential oil is often combined with clove oil to act as a painkiller and antiseptic when applied directly to toothaches. Cinnamon sticks are an essential ingredient in Indian chai tea, which soothes sore throats, coughs and colds. Cinnamon also stimulates the appetite while easing nausea and vomiting. Ayurvedic remedies for gas, hiccups and backache often include cinnamon.

Available forms

Cinnamon bark can be purchased in the form of sticks or powder. The sticks can be placed in a blender to obtain the strongest ground cinnamon. Cinnamon essential oil is also available from health food stores. A powerful remedy with cinnamon for respiratory conditions, Elatwagadi churnam is available from Ayurvedic clinics.

Home remedies

For a lovely warming tea at the onset of a cold, flu or cough, try the following recipe. Mix 2 cups of boiling water with the following ingredients:

- 2 cinnamon sticks;
- 2 cloves;
- 2 black peppercorns;
- 8 thin slices of ginger root (or 1 tsp grated ginger);
- 2 cardamom pods (slightly bruised); and
- 5 holy basil leaves.

Simmer the mixture, partially covered, for 10 minutes. Strain and add 1 tsp honey or palm sugar. Drink one cup three times a day.

Caution: If you are suffering from hemorrhaging, do not use cinnamon, as its heating properties can aggravate bleeding.

> *Cinnamon is sweet, bitter and decreases vata and pitta. It is a cooling and fragrant reproductive tonic that improves the complexion.*
> —Bhava Prakasha Samhita
> [An ancient Ayurvedic text]

Cloves

Syzygium aromaticum
Sanskrit: Lavangam **Hindi:** Lavanga
FAMILY: Myrtaceae

Cloves are renowned for their ability to ease respiratory ailments, aid low blood pressure, and alleviate impotence. Cloves help stop vomiting and will soothe the pain of toothache.

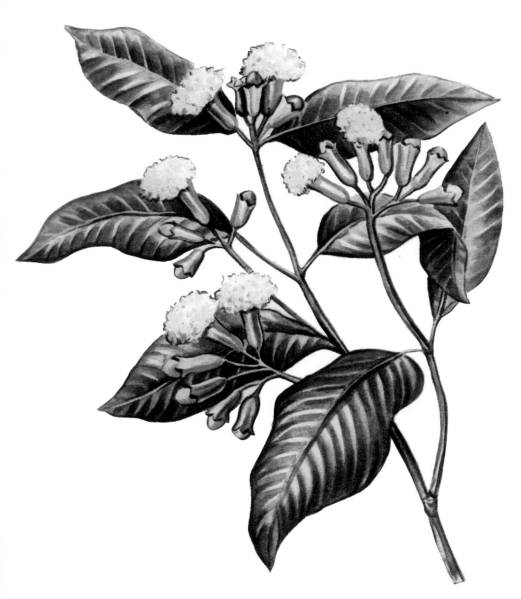

Description

Cloves are the dried, unopened flower buds of a tropical evergreen myrtle tree that grows best near the sea. The myrtaceous tree grows to 15–45 ft (5–14 m) and has elliptical leaves, gray bark, small, reddish-yellow flowers and purple fruit. The clove itself resembles a nail with a small head and a tapered shaft. It is thought that the name "clove" came from the Latin word for nail, "clavus." The tree grows in Madagascar, Sri Lanka, Brazil and Malaysia. Cloves were originally native to Indonesia.

Historical or mythological background

In ancient China, cloves were mentioned in documents dating back to 400 BC, and were used as a form of breath freshener by courtiers preparing to meet the Emperor. In Indonesia, the tree that produced cloves was considered sacred, and for each child born into the community, a tree was planted. It was believed that the fate of the child and the tree were intertwined, the tree symbolizing the child's development and state of health. Cloves were also used in love potions, and to enhance a person's psychic visions.

Modern uses

Traditionally employed as a respiratory and digestive tonic, cloves are valued in Ayurveda for their ability to cleanse toxins and mucus from the body. As an effective expectorant for

> *Clove flowers improve immunity, are cold in potency and cure pitta-related disorders. The auspicious clove improves eyesight, heals poisons and diseases of the head.*
> —Dhanwantari Nighantu
> *[An ancient Ayurvedic text]*

coughs and colds, cloves can be taken as an infusion, or the essential oil can be used in an inhalation. When the infection involves an increase in heat, rock sugar is combined with cloves to provide a cooling counterbalance. Cloves' stimulating quality is used to improve cases of low blood pressure and low libido.

Available forms

Health food stores sell clove essential oil for inhalation. Clove powder or whole clove is available from supermarkets or spice stores. One can find a fluid extract of clove from herbalists or selected health food stores. Twageladi churnam is a clove-rich traditional powder for respiratory and digestive problems available from most Ayurvedic clinics.

Home remedies

Wet a cotton ball in warm water and soak in 2 drops clove essential oil and 3 drops garlic oil. Place this on a toothache or tooth abscess to reduce pain and infection. Make a great gargle for sore throats by adding to 3 cups warm water the following ingredients:

- 5 drops tea tree oil;
- 3 drops clove oil;
- a pinch of turmeric powder;
- $^3/_4$ tsp–1 tsp rock salt or sea salt;
- 10 ml red sage tincture (optional); and
- 2 tbsps glycerin.

Mix all the ingredients well and gargle this twice daily until your symptoms subside.

Coriander

Coriandrum sativum, Coriander seeds, Cilantro
Sanskrit: Dhanyak **Hindi:** Dhania
FAMILY: Umbelliferae

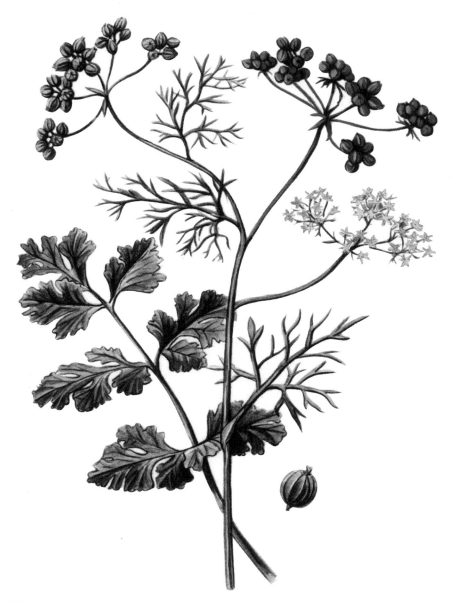

Coriander is an excellent tonic, aiding the digestion and easing the symptoms of respiratory problems such as allergies, sore throats and hay fever.

Description
Coriander is an annual plant that grows 1–2 ft (30–60 cm) high and has round, light-green stems. The leaves are light green, the root is white, spindly and slightly hairy, and the flowers are white with a reddish hue. The seeds, which are globular in shape and range from yellow to red to brown in color, are used for medicinal purposes. The plant grows in America, Morocco and Romania, and is common throughout India.

Historical or mythological background
Coriander has been known for many thousands of years, since at least 5000 BC. One of the earliest recordings of

coriander was from Sanskrit writings dated at around 1500 BC. It is even mentioned in the Bible (Exodus 16:31), in which "manna" is described as "white like Coriander Seed." Coriander has also been used as a protective herb—hung inside the house to protect it from negative energies and to attract harmony and peace. When grown in the garden, coriander is believed to protect the gardener and his or her family from harm.

Modern uses

Coriander is a favorite spice in Ayurvedic cooking, as it brings all three body types into balance. Both the seeds and the leaves are very cooling and cleansing. The leaf juice is rich in natural vitamin C and bioflavonoids, which strengthen the capillaries and blood vessels. This can be applied to the treatment of allergies, hay fever, rashes, varicose veins, piles and hemorrhaging. An infusion of the seeds eases eye disorders such as conjunctivitis and redness. Coriander's diuretic action helps to heal urinary tract infections and gout by clearing bacteria and nitrogenous waste from the kidneys and bladder. Seeds added to bean and vegetable dishes aid digestion and reduce gas. They also help to combat coughs, pharyngitis and sore throats.

Available forms

For the freshest coriander leaves, grow them in your garden or choose the greenest bunch from your local greengrocer or supermarket. Coriander seeds are stocked at most spice or grocery stores. Though ground coriander is readily available, it is much stronger when freshly ground with a spice or coffee grinder at home. A renowned Ayurvedic remedy for fever called shadanga kashayam contains coriander.

Home remedies

Coriander leaves contain natural antihistamines useful for combating allergic eye conditions such as hay fever. Try juicing 1 cup fresh coriander leaves with $1/3$ cup warm water, and drinking it on an empty stomach morning and evening to improve your digestion. To reduce nausea, gas and morning sickness, partially crush 4 tsp coriander seeds and combine with 2 tsp grated ginger. Boil this mixture in 4 cups water until it is reduced to 2 cups. Strain and drink one cup in the morning and afternoon.

Coriander is warming, pungent, sweet, fragrant and diuretic but doesn't increase pitta. Perfect as a culinary herb, it adds a flavor burst to every meal. It tones the vocal cords and cures burning sensations and thirst.
—Madanadi Nighantu
[An ancient Ayurvedic text]

Cumin

Cumin cyminum,
Sanskrit: Jiraka **Hindi:** Jira
FAMILY: Umbelliferae

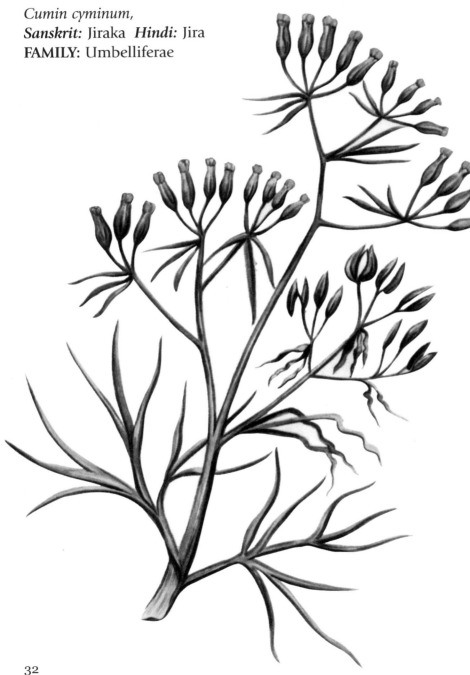

Cumin is one of the ancient spices. It has been used as a tonic and for digestive, anti-inflammatory and stimulant purposes.

Description

Cumin is an annual herb that grows to about 1 ft (30 cm). It has blue-green leaves, white or reddish-purple flowers and aromatic fruits that are grayish in color. These fruits turn pale green when dried, and are elliptical in shape, with deep ridges. The plant is native to the Levant, Upper Egypt and the Mediterranean. Although cumin is capable of adapting to a range of climates, it thrives best in warm, moist climates and in well-drained, sandy soil. The plant is cultivated in India, particularly in Gujarat, Rajasthan and Uttar Pradesh.

Historical or mythological background

Known since ancient times, cumin seeds were found in the Old Kingdom pyramids.

Cumin was prized during the time of the ancient Greeks and Romans for its medicinal properties and its cosmetic application for those seeking a pale complexion. The Roman scholar, Pliny the Elder (Gaius Plinius Secundus, 23–79AD), believed that ingestion of the spice would produce a studious scholar. Cumin was also used for good luck amulets, and a pinch of the spice each day was thought to encourage an active sex life.

Modern uses

Cumin shares similar healing properties with fennel and coriander. The seeds are included in almost every Ayurvedic meal, as they boost digestion and counter the gaseous effect of beans and potatoes. Cumin is often given with asafetida to reduce menstrual cramps and abdominal colic. Black cumin is the preferred variety for these conditions. Combined with fennel seeds, it is used to increase breast milk in nursing mothers. Cumin is also traditionally taken for diarrhea.

Available forms

Black and brown cumin seeds are sold at most Asian grocery stores and supermarkets. The powder can be ground at home from the seeds for the freshest flavor. Ayurvedic physicians often prescribe a warming wine—called *jirakarishtam*—as a uterine and digestive tonic.

> *All three types of cumin are dry, pungent, warm, digestive and light. They increase pitta, improve absorption and memory and cleanse the female reproductive system. Cumin is an antipyretic, digestive, carminative, fertility tonic and appetizer. It reduces kapha and vata, bloating, stomachaches, vomiting and diarrhea and strengthens the sight.*
> —Bhava Prakasha Samhita
> *[An ancient Ayurvedic text]*

Home remedies

Cooking with cumin is the easiest way to enjoy it's stomachic properties with every meal. Add $1/3$ tsp powder or $1/2$ tsp roasted seeds per serving to each dish. To overcome gassy indigestion or to perk up your appetite, mix the following ingredients together:

- 1 tsp cumin seeds;
- 1 tsp fennel seeds;
- $1/4$ tsp ground ginger; and
- $1/5$ tsp rock salt.

This mixture can be made into a tea by infusing it in hot water for 10 minutes and straining, or by simply chewing $1/2$ tsp of it 15 minutes before a meal. To relieve sinusitis, mix an equal quantity of ground holy basil, black pepper, black cumin seeds and turmeric. Take $1/3$ tsp two hours after breakfast and dinner with $1/4$ cup warm water.

Fennel

Foeniculum vulgaris, Fennel seeds
Sanskrit: Shatapushpa *Hindi:* Saumph
FAMILY: Umbelliferae

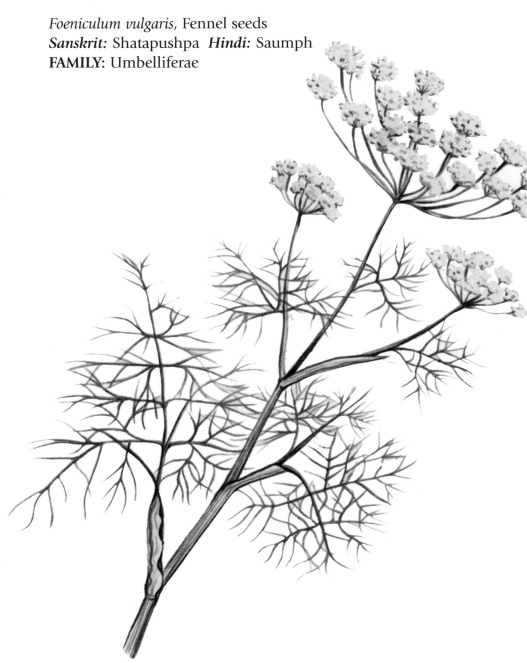

Fennel is an excellent antispasmodic herb, helpful for easing cramps and nausea. It also helps increase a weak appetite and relieves the buildup of mucus in the body.

Description

Fennel is a perennial plant that grows up to 4–5 ft (1.2–1.8 m). The stout stem grows from a carrot-shaped root. The plant has slim, pointed, feathery leaves and small, yellow flowers and elliptical fruits that are brown with a hint of yellow or green. The dried fruits are called seeds. The plant is native to the Mediterranean and is cultivated throughout India and in Egypt, the south of France and Russia. It thrives best in limestone soils situated in a dry and sunny place, but it also grows well in ordinary soil.

Historical or mythological background

In ancient times, fennel was believed to restore eyesight. Pliny the Elder (Gaius Plinius Secundus, 23–79AD) observed that snakes ate fennel when they were casting off their skins so as to restore their eyesight. This is reflected in the use, by Western practitioners, of fennel as an eye bath for eyestrain. The plant was considered a herb of protection for the house, and if gathered at midsummer's eve, a bunch was hung over every opening to the house. Fennel is also used for culinary purposes. It is best combined with cumin and coriander to produce a mixture of spices excellent for poor digestion without overstimulating the system.

Modern uses

Fennel is hailed as one of Ayurveda's best female tonics. It promotes menstruation and breast milk while

> *Fennel is a digestive, a taste enhancer and a mild laxative as well as being good for eliminating worms. The fruits are good for cough, vomiting, nausea and the disorders of kapha and vata.*
> —Madana Pala Nighantu
> *[An ancient Ayurvedic text]*

reducing menstrual cramps and premenstrual sugar cravings. Fennel is also a male aphrodisiac, increasing semen production. The seeds are chewed after meals to encourage digestion. Breastfeeding mothers can safely take an infusion of the seeds to pacify their babies' colic.

Available forms

One of the easiest ways to take fennel is in tea form, available from health food stores. The seeds and powder are also a tasty addition to many dishes, and are sold widely at most grocery stores or delicatessens. If you plant fennel bulbs in your garden, they are generally very hardy and fast-growing.

Home remedies

A cooling drink suitable to drink during the summer months and to alleviate pitta ailments, such as stomach ulcers, can be made by combining equal parts fennel seeds, mint leaves, lime, and cane sugar (sucanat) with a dash of rose water and a pinch of sandalwood powder. Serve in 10 parts cool purified water or coconut water. To reduce sugar cravings, particularly those that occur premenstrually, take a cup of fennel tea three times a day.

Caution: Fennel should only be taken under medical supervision during pregnancy, as it can stimulate uterine contractions.

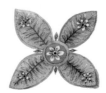

Frankincense (Indian)

Boswellia serrata
Sanskrit: Sallaki *Hindi:* Salai
FAMILY: Burseraceae

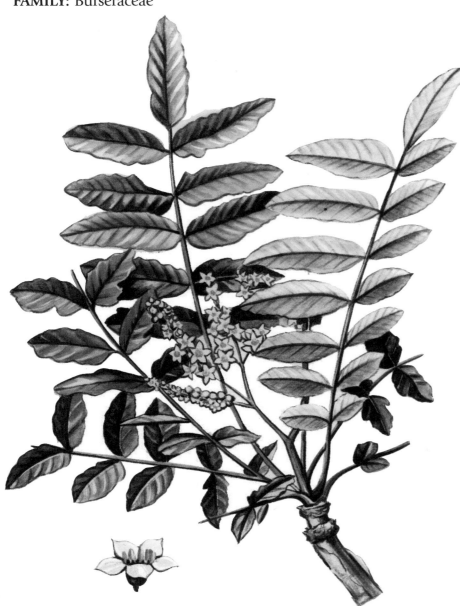

Frankincense has a calming effect and helps pacify fear and anxiety. It has also been used for pain relief and strengthening the nervous system.

Description

Indian frankincense is the resin that exudes from a deciduous tree with pale bark and small, white or pale rose-colored flowers. The color of the resin varies from golden to dark brown. The tree grows throughout central and northern India. These trees also grow in the south of Saudi Arabia and along the coastline of Somalia, where the trees grow without soil, clinging onto marble rocks. To collect the resin, the tree is cut and the resin is scraped from the cut when it has dried.

Historical or mythological background

Frankincense has been used since ancient times, becoming a popular ingredient for incense for religious ceremonies. In the New

Testament, it was one of the three gifts given to the infant Jesus. In Egypt, frankincense was one of the ingredients thrown onto a brazier warming a room; the kohl used by Egyptian women to highlight their eyelids was at one time made from charred frankincense. In China, frankincense was used to treat leprosy; the Romans also used the resin as incense. In the Middle Ages, frankincense was recommended for tumors, ulcers, vomiting, and fever. When used as an essential oil, frankincense is believed to be capable of removing negative energy and fears.

Modern uses
Ayurveda prescribes Indian frankincense extensively to treat autoimmune inflammatory conditions. These conditions include notoriously stubborn diseases such as ulcerative colitis, arthritis, psoriasis, and irritable bowel syndrome.

Indian and German studies have concluded that Indian frankincense gives significant improvement in cases of osteoarthritis, rheumatoid arthritis and chronic juvenile arthritis. Indian frankincense resin contains painkilling acids that also ease the discomfort of musculo-skeletal disorders. As a gargle, it helps reduce inflammation in sore throats, including tonsillitis. The antitumor and cholesterol-lowering activity of Indian frankincense has been helpful with skin tumors.

Available forms
Tablets and the fluid extracts of Indian frankincense (also known as Boswellia) are sold by most herbalists and health food stores. The concentrated resin is used in Ayurvedic dispensaries but is rarely taken alone. For specialty Ayurvedic combinations, contact your local Ayurvedic physician or distributor.

Home remedies
Indian frankincense has been shown to have very low toxicity, making it a relatively safe herb with which to experiment. Make the following juice to help reduce the pain and swelling of arthritis. Combine the following ingredients and drink them with one cup of water once a day on an empty stomach:

- a crushed tablet of 1.5 grams Indian frankincense resin;
- 2 cups fresh celery;
- a 2-inch (5 cm) slice of peeled ginger; and
- 1 gram Indian myrrh (guggulu).

Indian frankincense is bitter, sweet and astringent in taste; a powerful substance that improves absorption; alleviates blood disorders; balances vata and kapha; and cures dermatitis, hemorrhoids, ulcers and many painful conditions.
—Kayyadeva Nighantu
[An ancient Ayurvedic text]

Garlic

Allium sativum, Clove garlic, Poor man's treacle
Sanskrit: Rasona **Hindi:** Salai
FAMILY: Liliaceae

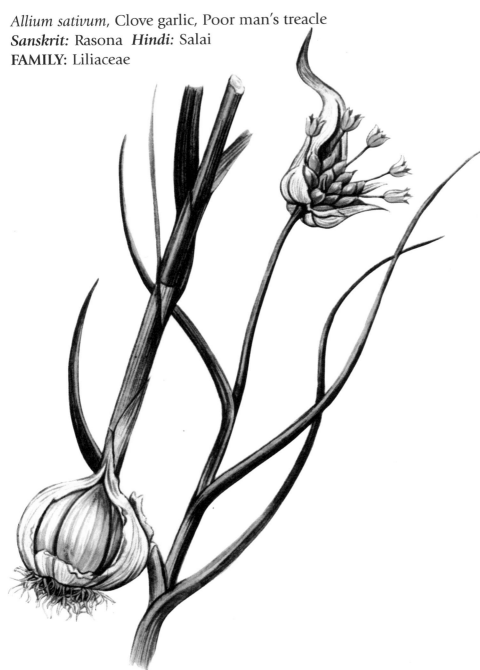

Garlic is an excellent cleanser of the blood and the nerves and has even been thought to ward off the "Evil Eye."

Description

The root of a perennial herb, garlic grows in a bulb that consists of a number of cloves, each covered with a papery, white skin. Additional layers of skin also form an outer covering for a number of cloves, holding them together into a bulb. A round stem rises from the center of the bulb, which is encased with leaf sheaths. The stem ends in a spike within which grow small, white flowers that are tinged with purple. The plant is native to central Asia and flourishes best when it is in a sunny location and planted in rich, moist, sandy soil.

Historical or mythological background

Garlic has a very long history of use for both culinary and medicinal purposes. It is believed that its use dates back more than 5,000 years. A wide range of civilizations, from the Greeks and Romans to the Vikings and the Egyptians, have recorded using garlic. In Egypt, about 2600 BC, garlic was given to the workers who were building the Great Pyramid at Giza because the herb was considered to be excellent for strengthening and for warding off disease. Garlic has also had a reputation for being able to ward off the "Evil Eye."

Modern uses

Garlic's powerful antibiotic action makes it an irreplaceable panacea in Ayurveda's apothecary. Known as an immune stimulant (rasayana), its sulphurous compounds are preventative against infections such as earaches, coughs, pneumonia, colds and septic wounds. Garlic reduces cholesterol, which in turn reduces the risk of heart attacks and strokes. It also lowers blood pressure and reduces blood clotting. Garlic has versatile uses in digestive disorders, as it increases the appetite as well as liquefying and expelling toxins.

Available forms

Fresh garlic cloves are generally more potent than deodorized garlic, as much of garlic's medicinal properties are contained in its odor. However, naturally aged garlic can be odorless while still retaining its therapeutic value. Concentrated garlic oil, tablets and fluid extracts are available from most supermarkets and are always stocked in health food stores.

Home remedies

The early stages of earaches and infections can be treated with garlic and onion oil. Warm 1 tbsp olive oil in a pan over a low flame and add to it 2 garlic cloves and 1 tsp chopped onion that have been crushed in a garlic press. Heat on a low flame for 5 minutes, then take off the stove to settle for 5 minutes. Strain the mixture, and use 2 ml of the resulting oil in the affected ear twice daily.

Caution: garlic should be taken with caution in pitta conditions, especially with bleeding and rashes, and during pregnancy and breastfeeding.

> *When a demon called Rahu stole the nectar from the gods, a few drops dropped onto earth, transforming into garlic. Hence Yogis don't eat garlic, because it came from a demon. However Ayurveda considers it to be the supreme rejuvenator.*
> —Ashtanga Hrdayam
> *[An ancient book on Ayurvedic healing]*

Ginger

Zingiber officinale, African ginger
Sanskrit: Sunthi *Hindi:* Adarak
FAMILY: Zingiberaceae

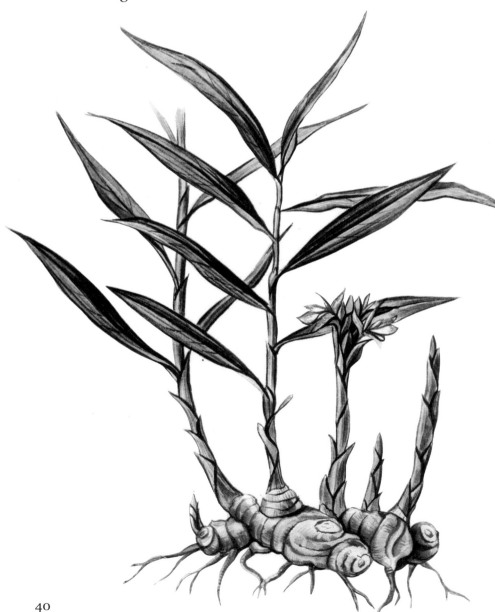

As a digestive, ginger eases abdominal cramping, nausea and vomiting, and, as an expectorant, it is extremely useful in combating colds.

Description

Ginger is the root of a perennial plant from which a green, reed-like stalk grows to 2–3 ft (60–90 cm) high. From the stalk, long, thin, pointed leaves grow. The stalk ends with a spike from which emerge yellow flowers or white ones with purple tinges. The root is thick and light brown in color. Inside, the root is fibrous, juicy and yellow. Ginger was first grown in Asia and thrives in tropical climates. It is cultivated in the West Indies, Jamaica and India.

Historical or mythological background

The use of ginger has been known for many centuries, the plant featuring in the medical literature of the ancient

Greeks, Romans and Arabs. The Chinese and Indians first cultivated ginger. The word "ginger" came from a Sanskrit word "sringivera," meaning "shaped like a horn." The yogis believed that ginger enhanced mental clarity; as it left a fresh scent in the mouth, it was very popular among the yogis, as it did not offend the gods. The state of the ginger plant growing in a garden was believed to be symbolic of the state of the gardener's health.

Modern uses

Ginger's diverse repertoire of uses has earned it the title of *vishwabesaj* or "universal medicine." Both Ayurvedic

> *Ginger balances diseases related to kapha and vata. It also cures blockages of various kinds, bloating, pains and infertility. It is a pungent, hot appetizer also good for improving immunity.*
> —Raja Nighantu
> *[An ancient Ayurvedic text]*

and Chinese herbalists use it in over 80 percent of their formulas, aiding the distribution and assimilation of the accompanying herbs. Chewing on raw ginger root or drinking a strong infusion often alleviates nausea due to morning sickness or motion sickness. Internally, it is an effective remedy for colds, flu, cough, and poor circulation. Combined with black pepper and long pepper, it is a favorite Ayurvedic compound called trikatu, useful for flatulence and poor digestion. Its addition as a culinary herb in most Asian dishes promotes digestion by stimulating digestive secretions. Externally, a ginger poultice is soothing for arthritis, lumbago, kidney pain and sciatica.

Available forms

Fresh ginger and dried ginger have very similar effects, but fresh ginger is a little more pungent and drying in the body than dried ginger. Plentiful at most grocery stores, fresh ginger is more palatable with the skin removed.

Home remedies

Manage the trials of travel sickness by chewing a slice of ginger root every hour, or sip a strong cup of ginger root tea during the journey. To improve circulation, a tea of cinnamon, pepper and ginger is excellent. Combine 2 cinnamon sticks with 5 thin slices ginger and one peppercorn in 2 cups water. Boil down to $1\frac{1}{2}$ cups. Strain the mixture and let it cool. Drink it twice daily, an hour before meals.

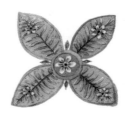

Gooseberry (Indian)

Ribes grossularia, Emblica officinalis
Sanskrit: Amalaki *Hindi:* Amla
FAMILY: Grossulariaceae

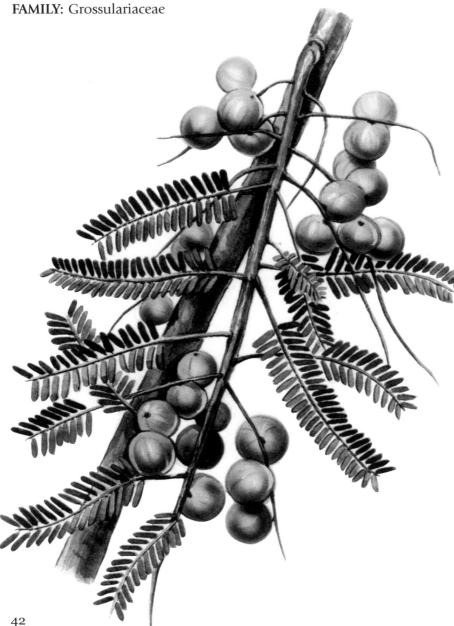

Indian gooseberry is a useful tonic, very high in Vitamin C content, and is famous for its sedative qualities.

Description
Indian gooseberry is a tropical deciduous tree that grows up to 3–4 ft (1–1.2 m) high. It has feathery leaves and smooth, grayish-green bark with globular, fleshy fruits. The fruits, which are a berry, are sour in taste and contain a number of small seeds at the center. There are over 200 varieties of gooseberry. The European gooseberry grows in central and northern Europe. The Indian gooseberry is found in deciduous forests that grow up to an altitude of 4,500 ft (1,500 m). Gooseberry also grows in Nepal, Morocco and America.

Historical or mythological background
Indian gooseberry has been used in Ayurvedic medicine for over 5,000 years, featuring in

such medicinal preparations as *triphala* (a rejuvenative/laxative) and *chyavanaprasham* (a tonic to promote mental and physical well-being). These trees are also the dwelling place for a number of deities in south Indian villages, including Shiva, Subrahmanya and Vishnu. Indian gooseberry is believed to calm mothers who are angry with their children, and to help children feel nurtured if they have been deprived of their mothers.

Modern uses

Gooseberry's nurturing and curative reputation has earned it the title of "the nurse." It balances all three doshas, but is especially helpful for pitta disorders, which include

Gooseberries are the safest for healing and balancing all aggravated doshas.
—Rajavallabha Nighantu
[An ancient Ayurvedic text]

hemorrhaging, anemia, gastritis, premature graying, urinary tract infections, acidity and intermittent fevers. As each fruit contains about 3,000 mg of vitamin C, gooseberry is Ayurveda's principal antioxidant and immune stimulant. Gooseberry's cleansing action is used to strengthen the eyes, colon and teeth. It also helps to regulate blood sugar levels by optimizing liver, pancreas and spleen function.

Available forms

Gooseberry's astringent properties are most potent when taken as a raw fruit or in powder form. The pure tablets and powder are available at some health food stores, herbalists and Ayurvedic outlets. The shiny green fruits are rarely available outside Asia, but you may occasionally find the fresh fruit at some Chinese and Indian grocery stores. Preparations with a high proportion of

gooseberry, such as triphala and chyavanaprasham, are commonly sold at Indian grocery stores.

Home remedies

Triphala, or the "three fruits," a formula made with equal quantities of gooseberries, haritaki (*Terminalia chebula*) and vibhitaki (*Terminalia belerica*), is one of Ayurveda's best digestive and immune tonics. Gooseberry, by balancing the body's organs and systems, is useful for innumerable conditions. Taking $1\frac{1}{2}$ tsp before bed ensures a complete cleansing bowel movement the following morning. For eye disorders, ranging from glaucoma to irritation and redness, triphala eyewash generally offers noticeable relief. Place 1 heaped tsp triphala powder in hot water and cover overnight. In the morning, strain the mixture through a thin cloth and use the remaining liquid as an eyebath.

Licorice

Glycyrrhiza glabra, Licorice root, Sweet licorice, Sweetwood
Sanskrit: Yastimadhu *Hindi:* Jetimad
FAMILY: Leguminosae

Licorice is one of the best herbs for treating respiratory ailments. It is useful as an expectorant and is soothing for sore throats.

Description

Licorice is a perennial shrub with a stem that grows up to 2–5 ft (0.6–1.6 m) tall. The plant has narrow, long, dark-green leaves, yellowish-white or purple flowers, small, oblong pods and a brown legume fruit. The root and lower underground stems, which are left unpeeled and then dried, are the only parts of the plant used medicinally. Licorice is native to southern Europe, Asia and the Mediterranean and is cultivated in India, in the Punjab and the sub-Himalayan tracts. Licorice is also cultivated in Russia, Spain and Iran. It grows best in a dry, warm climate, thriving in sandy, rich soil.

History or mythological background

Licorice has been used in Ayurvedic medicine for many centuries, particularly for the treatment of upper respiratory ailments. The Egyptians first recorded using licorice in the 3rd century BC and, in the 1st century AD, Greek physician Dioscorides named the plant Glycyrrhiza from the Greek "glukos" meaning "sweet" and "riza" meaning "a root." In India, licorice is known as yastimadhu, a combination of yasti, meaning stick, and madhu, meaning sweet. In China, the herb is also very popular, used for the treatment of the spleen, liver and kidney.

Modern uses

The sweet, soothing effect of licorice makes it a popular addition to many Ayurvedic respiratory and digestive tonics. Commonly given for respiratory tract disorders, licorice eases the symptoms of laryngitis, asthma, bronchitis,

Licorice is sweet, cold, moist and heavy; improves the complexion and voice; is a tonic for the hair and fertility as well as being generally nourishing. It balances vata, pitta and kapha; healing wounds, nausea, vomiting, fatigue, edema and ulcers.
—Kayyadeva Nighantu
[An ancient Ayurvedic text]

colds, mouth ulcers and flu. As a digestive, it reduces acidity, heals gastric ulcers and acts as a mild laxative. A unique action is its ability to increase the production of anti-inflammatory hydrocortisone, which eases joint aches, asthma and skin conditions such as eczema. It also tonifies the adrenals, hastening recovery from stress or steroid use.

Available forms

Bad news for licorice addicts—confectionery licorice rarely contains one iota of the real stuff. However, laxative licorice pellets are sold at select health food stores and some pharmacies. Licorice powder and pure licorice root is stocked by Chinese and Ayurvedic herbalists. Fluid extracts, tea bags and tincture of licorice can be obtained from most health food stores or herbalists.

Home remedies

Licorice gives rapid relief at the initial signs of a sore throat. A tea can be made with 1 tsp each of licorice root, raw wild cherry bark, dry red sage, golden seal powder, ginger powder and 1/4 tsp trikatu. Add to 3 cups boiling water, then simmer down to 2 cups. Stir in some honey if desired. Strain and drink 2 cups three times a day.

Caution: Pregnant women and people suffering from high blood pressure or water retention should use licorice cautiously because it increases sodium retention.

Lotus

Nelumbo nucifera, Sacred lotus, Indian lotus, Chinese water lily
Sanskrit: Padma, Kamala, Pushkara, Shatapatra **Hindi:** Kamal
FAMILY: Nymphaeceae

The most sacred plant of India, the lotus is an important ingredient for rejuvenating the mind, body and spirit. It is also a useful digestive, aphrodisiac and tonic.

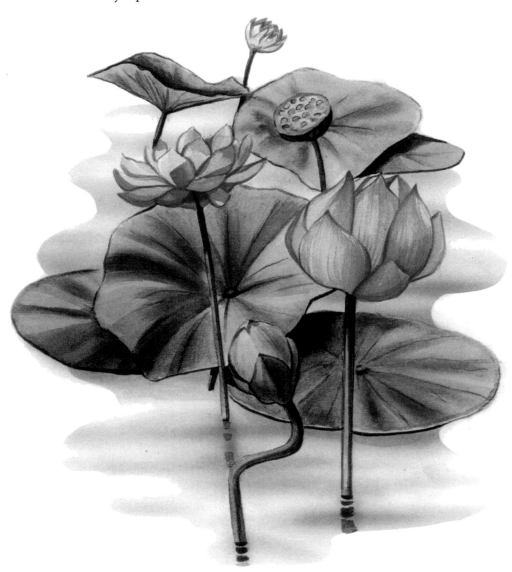

Description

The lotus is an aquatic herb with large, circular, leathery leaves measuring about 20 inches (50 cm) in diameter. The overall height of the plant is 3–6 ft (1–2 m). The leaves and large, fragrant, white or pink flowers with a yellow center float on the water. Slender, elongated roots reach down into, and fan out through, the mud of the pond. The flowers are solitary and the plant has many-seeded ovoid fruits. The lotus grows in shallow ponds and marshland throughout India up to an altitude of 5,400 ft (1,800 m).

Historical or mythological background

The lotus is the national flower of India, and in Indian mythology, it is sacred to the goddess of prosperity, Lakshmi. Lakshmi, the wife of Lord Vishnu, epitomizing female beauty, is often depicted sitting on a lotus. The Lord of Creation, Brahma, is also associated with the lotus. He is usually shown being born on a lotus sprouting from Lord Vishnu's navel. The lotus root and seeds have been used for devotional practices as the plant is believed to improve the mind's ability to focus and to encourage the development of a person's spirituality. The lotus is considered a metaphor for the soul, rooted in the mud of the material world but transcending limitations to rise toward the spiritual sky.

Modern uses

Ayurveda uses all parts of the lotus for different regions of the body. Since the seeds are high in protein, they encourage hormonal harmony. They are used as an aphrodisiac, for chronic diarrhea, for high blood pressure and fevers. The lotus roots increase sperm production, arrest bleeding and assist respiratory conditions such as pharyngitis. Lotus flowers are considered a tonic for the heart, liver and skin, particularly when aggravated pitta is involved. The leaves reduce fever, dizziness and headaches.

Available forms

Lotus leaves, stamens and petals are generally sold only by Chinese or Ayurvedic herbalists. However, the seeds, which contain much of the lotus's medicinal properties, are found at Asian grocery stores. In Chinese, they are known as *Lian zi*. These can be ground into powder for the most effective absorption.

> *Lotus is cooling, promoting sweat, and cures diseases of kapha and pitta, such as burning sensations and inflammatory skin conditions.*
> 6+Bhavaprakasha Nighantu
> *[An ancient Ayurvedic text]*

Home remedies

For women suffering from infertility, mix 1 tsp each of lotus root powder and shatavari powder with 1/4 cup aloe vera juice and 1/2 cup warm water. Drink this mixture twice a day on an empty stomach. As a reproductive tonic to boost sperm count and libido, combine in one cup of warm almond milk one hour before bed:

- 3 grams lotus seed powder;
- 3 grams lotus root powder;
- 5 grams Indian ginseng;
- 2 grams American ginseng; and
- honey to taste (optional).

Marshmallow

Althaea officinalis, Sweet weed, Schloss tea, Althea
FAMILY: Malvaceae

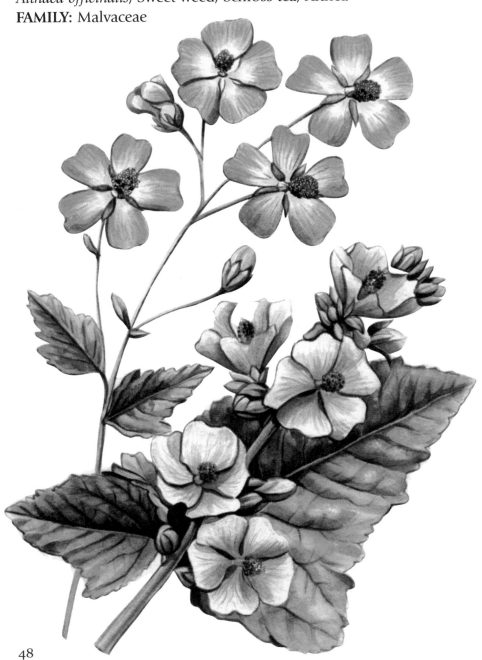

Used since ancient times, marshmallow is an excellent tonic and is soothing for both internal and external inflammations.

Description

Marshmallow is a sprawling, perennial and annual plant that grows about 3–4 ft (1–1.2 m) high. Its root is long, cream-colored, tapering and fibrous. The plant has a furry stem with large pointed and heart-shaped leaves covered with a velvety down. The plant also has pale pink flowers, which are followed by fruits (historically called "cheese" because of their resemblance to small rounds of flattened cheese). The plant grows mostly wild, usually in marshes, but is easily cultivated when planted in well-drained soil.

Historical or mythological background

The Romans used marshmallow as a general tonic; Pliny the Elder (Gaius Plinius Secundus, 23–79AD) believed that marshmallow could cure all the diseases of man. Early Ayurvedic physicians extolled its virtues as an anti-inflammatory, both for the respiratory and digestive tracts. Marshmallow's family name, Malvaceae, comes from the Greek *malake*, "to soften," which refers to its ability to soften hardened mucus.

Modern uses

Marshmallow's Greek name is "altho," meaning to heal. This herb is especially soothing to the mucous membranes of the digestive, respiratory and urinary tracts. It calms inflammatory disorders such as urinary tract infections, ulcers, laryngitis and bronchitis. In these conditions, it is often combined with bala (*Sida rhombifolia*) and slippery elm, a bark that has similar properties to marshmallow. Externally, combined with antiseptic herbs, it makes an excellent poultice for chronic ulcers, boils and infected wounds.

Available Forms

Dried marshmallow is sold at health food stores, and can be boiled into a decoction or infusion, or made into a poultice. The fluid extract and ointment are also available from health food stores, but avoid the ones made with petroleum-based emulsions, as this interferes with marshmallow's soothing and healing effects.

Home remedies

To restore an inflamed respiratory or digestive tract, the following marshmallow-based tea is a time-tested remedy. Combine the following ingredients and boil them in 4 cups water until the liquid is reduced to 3 cups:

- 10 grams marshmallow herb;
- 3 grams licorice root powder;
- 10 grams bala powder; and
- a pinch of ginger powder.

Strain the tea and stir in 1 tsp slippery elm powder. Drink one cup three times daily.

To make a poultice for ulcers, boils or wounds, combine equal quantities of marshmallow leaves, comfrey, golden seal powder and slippery elm powder. Add enough water to make a thick paste. Apply the poultice to the affected area, covering it with a lightly steamed or bruised cabbage leaf and a cloth soaked in warm water. Keep the cloth warm by dipping in warm water as required. Continue this procedure for 20–30 minutes. If there is a severe infection, mix some neem powder or turmeric powder into the poultice. After removing the poultice, spray the area with a very diluted solution of neem seed extract, tea tree oil and turmeric water.

Myrrh

Commiphora mukul
Sanskrit: Gugguluh **Hindi:** Guggul
FAMILY: Burseraceae

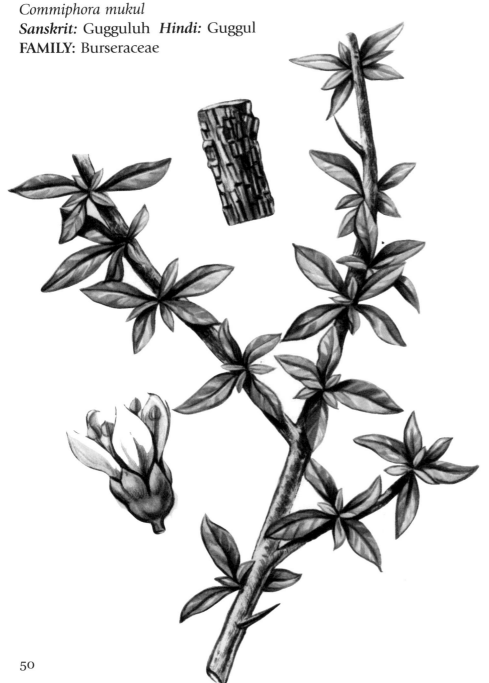

Indian myrrh has been used for centuries as an ingredient in incense and perfumes and is an excellent tonic with astringent and healing qualities.

Description

Myrrh is a gum resin collected from the stem of a bush that grows up to 9 ft (3 m) in height. The bush features small, oval leaves, and grows in the rocky regions of Rajasthan as well as in Gujarat, Assam and Bangladesh. A pale-yellow gum is secreted from ducts in the bark surrounding the stem. When the gum has hardened into an opaque, deep brown–red color, the resin is collected. The resin is usually quite brittle, with a powdery surface.

Historical or mythological background

Myrrh has been an important part of ancient practices in Muslim, Jewish and Christian religions. The ancient Egyptians used myrrh in their embalming and fumigating procedures. The resin was used for thousands of years in Middle Eastern medicine to heal cuts and wounds and to alleviate the symptoms of bronchitis. In Ayurvedic medicine, myrrh was used for its astringent qualities and formed the base for toothpowder and mouthwash. The resin was introduced to the Chinese and the Tibetans in the 7th century AD.

Modern uses

Indian myrrh is Ayurveda's primary weight-loss and cholesterol-lowering herb. Recent studies reveal that it stimulates thyroid function. This in turn lowers cholesterol and raises the metabolism, facilitating weight loss. Its anti-inflammatory and painkilling action makes it a favorite remedy for arthritic and rheumatic conditions. Since Indian myrrh is also an excellent blood purifier, it is used to overcome many toxic states such as liver disease, menstrual disorders, diabetes and skin imbalances. It can also be used as a nerve tonic and painkiller.

Available forms

When looking for Indian myrrh (also known as guggul), be careful not to buy common myrrh instead. All Ayurvedic outlets sell Indian myrrh or guggulu tablets, powder, decoctions and jams, as it is a staple herb for any dispensary. Combinations such as mahayoggaraja guggul tablets for arthritis or kaishora guggulu tablets for urinary-tract problems may target your specific needs more effectively than plain guggulu.

Home remedies

For the pain of arthritis or inflammatory nerve conditions such as sciatica, warm 1 tbsp castor oil on a low heat and add ½ tsp Indian myrrh powder plus ⅓ tsp ginger powder. Stir well and take it off the heat after a few minutes. Massage gently into the affected region. Leave this on for at least one hour and at most eight hours. For high cholesterol or obesity, take ⅓ tsp Indian myrrh powder with ½ tsp triphala powder twice a day on an empty stomach.

Guggulu is fragrant, light, subtle, intense, hot and pungent. A tonic for the heart, it improves the flow in all channels. Fresh guggulu is a tonic and improves fertility. Old guggulu is a strong anti-lipid substance. Guggulu balances kapha and vata with its intense and hot qualities, cures pitta and toxins with its moistness and improves the metabolic fire with its penetrative nature.
Sushruta Samhita
[An ancient Ayurvedic text]

Neem

Azadirachta indica
Sanskrit: Nimba, Prabhadrah **Hindi:** Neem
English: Neem tree
FAMILY: Meliaceae

Neem is renowned for its protective qualities, both spiritually and medically. A powerful detoxifier, neem is particularly effective for cleansing the blood, which aids skin ailments.

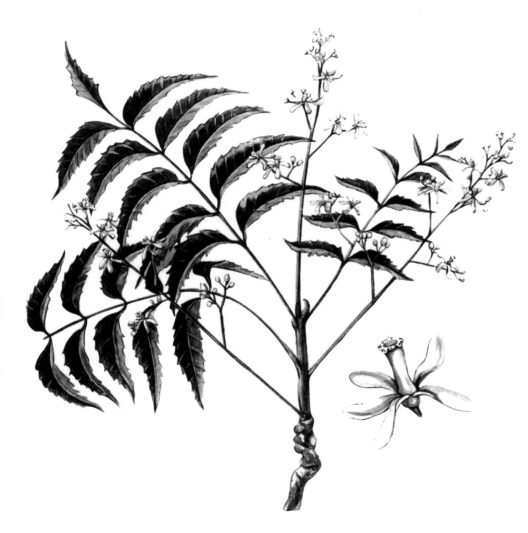

Description

Neem is a tropical evergreen tree that grows to a height of 45–60 ft (15–20 m). The tree has brown to dark-gray bark and small flowers that grow in clusters. The flowers are white or cream in color. It is a lush-looking tree with pinnate leaves; its roots bury deep into the soil. Its fruit, which is greenish-yellow in color when ripe, contains one seed that is elliptical and oily. Neem is native to India, growing in most soil types up to an elevation of 5,400 ft (1,800 m). It is cultivated in tropical, subtropical, and semi-arid areas in Africa, South East Asia, the Caribbean, Fiji and Australia.

Historical or mythological background

The Sanskrit name for neem, "nimba," is derived from the phrase "nimbati swastyamdadati', which means "to give good health." Neem has been used in Ayurvedic medicine since ancient times, when it was called "sarva roga nivarini" (the cure of all ills). The sacred quality of the neem tree is derived from a number of Indian myths, including the legend of Indra, the king of heaven, who spilled a drop of amrita (the nectar of immortality) onto a neem tree, imbuing it with magical healing powers. It is believed that if three neem trees are planted in the garden, the owner of the garden will be protected from going to hell.

Modern uses

Neem is a powerful blood purifier. It aids in the treatment of skin problems such as eczema, psoriasis, acne, ringworm and

Neem is bitter, cold, light and reduces kapha, blood and pitta related disorders. It cures dermatitis, pruritus and ulcers with internal or external usage. It has the power to digest toxins and eliminate diseased tissues.
—Dhanwantari Nighantu [An ancient Ayurvedic text]

boils, and is also used as a preventative against infections such as malaria, measles, chickenpox and hepatitis. It is also an effective insect repellant. Ayurvedic practitioners claim that a few neem leaves a day will keep the worms away. By boosting liver, spleen and pancreas function, neem is a tonic for liver diseases and diabetes.

Available forms

For external use, neem soap, shampoo, nit wash, cleanser, acne gel and seed-oil extract are available through shops, markets or the Internet. Ayurvedic clinics and suppliers sell neem powder, tablets and decoctions. Growing a hardy neem tree in your yard helps to keep insects away, nourishes the soil and provides easy access to its healing leaves. For the adventurous, the frayed end of a neem twig is a traditional toothbrush.

Home remedies

Neem is one of Ayurveda's strongest anti-fungal herbs. To treat tinea, ringworm or any fungal skin condition, apply pure neem-seed oil to the affected area twice daily. This can be combined with $1/4$ tsp concentrated tea tree oil and $1/5$ tsp turmeric powder for stubborn conditions. To purify the blood and colon of bacteria, fungus or parasites, take 1 tsp neem leaf powder in $1/4$ cup warm water 1 hour before meals twice daily.

Pepper (Long)

Piper longum, Indian long pepper
Sanskrit: Pippali *Hindi:* Pipli
FAMILY: Piperaceae

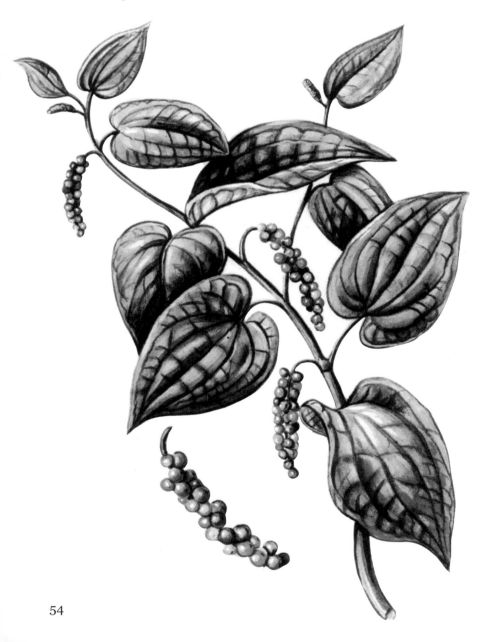

Indian long pepper is an excellent tonic for the lungs and helps cleanse mucus from the respiratory and digestive tracts. It is also an aphrodisiac that strengthens the reproductive organs.

Description

Indian long pepper is a slender climber with heart-shaped leaves. Solitary, cylindrical spikes flower opposite the leaves. The spikes are covered with ovoid fruits or berries that turn red when ripe. The unripe spikes are dried and used medicinally. The plant is grown in the central Himalayas, Assam and the forests of the western Ghats. The Indian long pepper is closely related to black pepper. Black pepper is native to southwestern India and is cultivated in China and Indonesia.

Historical or mythological background

Pepper has been used for both culinary and medicinal purposes for over 4,000 years. Long pepper was used well before black pepper became popular. However, in Ayurvedic medicine, black and long pepper are combined to make trikatu, which has powerful rejuvenative and digestive qualities. In China, pepper is used to treat digestive and liver disorders; it was believed that chewing the whole corn would increase physical stamina.

Modern uses

Long pepper is a warming digestive herb often combined with ginger and black pepper to create a treasured Ayurvedic digestive called trikatu. Most suited to excess vata conditions, long pepper increases the appetite, stimulates digestive enzymes, reduces gas and liquefies intestinal toxins.

It is often taken with other herbs, as it facilitates their optimal absorption and distribution in the body. For respiratory problems, long pepper expels and dries up mucus and dilates the bronchial passages, providing relief for such conditions as asthma, bronchitis, colds and laryngitis. Long pepper's ability to flush toxins from the joints and reduce pain is utilized in the treatment of arthritis, rheumatism, sciatica and gout. Because of its intensely pungent nature, long pepper should be used with caution in high pitta states.

Available forms

Long pepper is rarely given alone, but is generally prescribed in a combination either to buffer its extremely pungent nature or to aid its circulation throughout the body. The powdered combination called trikatu for respiratory and digestive conditions contains equal parts of black pepper, ginger and long pepper and is available from select health food stores and Ayurvedic herbal outlets. A traditional wine—called pippaliasavam— is a powerful digestive boost after meals.

Home remedies

To make your own trikatu, combine equal parts of powdered dried ginger, long pepper and black pepper. To treat colds, coughs or sore throats, take $1/3$ tsp in honey and $1/5$ cup water three times a day after or between meals. For indigestion, loss of appetite or gas, combine $1/3$ tsp trikatu with $1\frac{1}{2}$ tsp warm water half an hour before meals.

> Long pepper is anti-inflammatory, a fertility tonic, moist, warm, pungent and bitter. It is digestive and cures vata, kapha, dyspnea, cough and depletion.
> —Raja Nighantu
> [An ancient Ayurvedic text]

Pomegranate

Punica granatum
Sanskrit: Dadima *Hindi:* Anar
FAMILY: Punicaceae

Pomegranate is a useful digestive that has been associated with fertility and fruitfulness since ancient times.

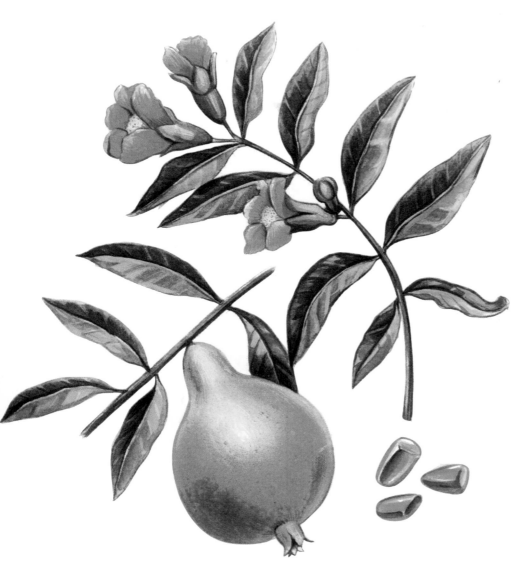

Description

The pomegranate is the fruit of a deciduous tree that grows to 12–16 ft (4–5 m). The tree has a bark-covered trunk that is red–brown to dark gray in color. It also has leathery, long, narrow leaves, scarlet or white flowers, and round or globular fruits that are often rich red in color. The pomegranate fruit has a leathery skin that breaks open easily when ripe to reveal an interior that is separated into compartments by membranous walls and white rind. Each compartment has a seed surrounded by sacs of juicy reddish pulp. The plant is native to the area between Iran and the Himalayas in north India. It is widely cultivated throughout India and in the drier parts of South

East Asia, the East Indies and Africa.

Historical or mythological background

Pomegranate has been cultivated since ancient times. Ayurvedic practitioners have used its roots, seeds and fruits as an astringent, as a digestive, and as a purgative to expel worms. It has been associated with fertility and fruitfulness. The ancient Greeks believed that the number of seeds that tumble out of a pomegranate thrown on the ground is an indication of how many children the person who has thrown the fruit will have. The fruit is also a symbol of abundance and has been incorporated into royal emblems or badges, such as the one for Catherine of Aragon and the decoration of King Solomon's Temple.

> *Moist, warm Pomegranate improves immunity and balances vata without agitating kapha and pitta.*
> Dhanwantari Nighantu
> *[An ancient Ayurvedic text]*

Modern uses

Apart from being a refreshing fruit, pomegranate has potent tonic and purifying properties. The fruit juice is a popular drink in India, especially during summer, as it cools the body while increasing red blood cell production and lowering acidity. The juice's astringent action helps alleviate the symptoms of diarrhea, indigestion, biliousness and bleeding disorders. The seeds and rind help to kill and expel worms, especially tapeworms, as well as healing colitis and ulcers. They are also used as a tonic for the heart, spleen and liver. Pomegranate's bark is also renowned for strengthening the gums.

Available forms

Powders, tablets, ghees and decoctions are all sold through Ayurvedic and some Chinese outlets. To enjoy the fresh fruit, look for it in large fruit and vegetable stores.

Home remedies

To boost your iron levels and to cleanse the colon, try a cup of fresh pomegranate juice with 1 tsp lime juice on an empty stomach first thing in the morning. Dadimashtaka churna is an Ayurvedic powder compound that combats diarrhea and dysentery. Combine the following ingredients:

- 1 tsp ajwan seed powder;
- 1 tsp ground cumin;
- 1 tsp coriander powder;
- 1 tsp trikatu;
- 8 tsp ground pomegranate rind; and
- 8 tsp palm sugar.

After stirring well, take $3/4$ tsp twice a day between meals with buttermilk, rice water or warm water.

Sandalwood

Santalum album, Sandal tree, white-sandal tree
Sanskrit: Chandana **Hindi:** Safed candan, Santal
FAMILY: Piperaceae

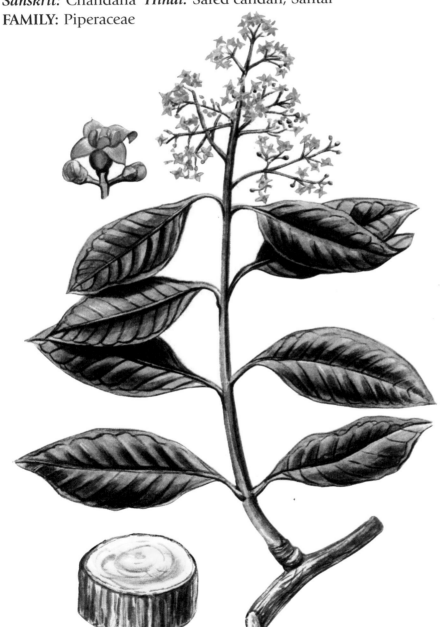

Sandalwood beans exude an aromatic oil that helps reduce fevers and inflammations and can be applied externally to ease infectious skin diseases.

Description

Sandalwood refers to both the wood and the oil taken from the sandal tree. The tree is an evergreen that grows to 54 ft (18 m) in height. Its branches droop from a trunk covered in bark. The bark is dark gray or brown–black, the leaves are oval, the flowers are purple and the fruits are globular and dark purple in color. The wood is very aromatic, straight-grained and, when first cut from the trunk of the tree, is white or yellow–brown in color. When dry, the wood turns dark brown with a reddish tinge. The tree grows primarily in India, preferring the dry regions of Karnataka, Tamilnadu and Kerala.

Historical or mythological background

Because of its cooling and calming qualities, sandalwood has been used in meditation practices. When applied to the third eye, which is the point in the middle of the forehead, it is believed that the feelings of heat or fever will abate. Burning oil or incense containing sandalwood is also believed to enhance the intelligence and sense of devotion experienced by a person practicing meditation. Combined with the mud of the Ganges River, the resulting sandalwood and mud paste is used to create tilak—religious markings on the body to designate it as the temple of the soul.

Modern uses

The wood and volatile oil of sandalwood is a virtual panacea for extreme pitta ailments, such as sunstroke. As a strong antibacterial, antiviral and antiseptic agent, it helps to combat urinary tract infections, gonorrhea, herpes zoster and skin infections. Eyedrops containing sandalwood reduce burning, stinging and inflamed eyes. The cooling powder can also relieve fevers and thirst.

Available forms

Since sandalwood is a protected species, its export is restricted. This means it can be difficult to get pure sandalwood powder outside of Asia. The best place to look for it is at Hindu temples, Indian shops and Ayurvedic clinics. However, pure sandalwood incense is the next best thing to the pure powder.

> *All types of sandalwoods are bitter and pungent in taste. Extremely cold in potency, they improve fertility and tone the heart. They are fragrant and cure blood and pitta related diseases such as bleeding conditions.*
> —Bhava Prakasha Samhita
> *[An ancient Ayurvedic text]*

Home remedies

A simple and highly effective beauty mask used in India for centuries has sandalwood powder as its base. Mix together the following ingredients:

- 12 parts fine chickpea flour;
- 3 parts sandalwood powder;
- 2 parts neem leaf powder; and
- 1 part turmeric powder.

Take 1 tbsp of this combination and add enough water to make a thick cream. Apply to problem areas, leaving it on for 10 minutes. Clean off with a cold washcloth and follow with a rose-water toner. For a lovely cooling drink in summer, a pinch of sandalwood powder can be added to 1 cup pure water with 2 tsp finely chopped fresh mint leaves.

Sarsaparilla (Indian)

Hemidesmus indicus
Sanskrit: Anantamula, Sariba **Hindi:** Anantumul, Magrabu
FAMILY: Asclepiadaceae

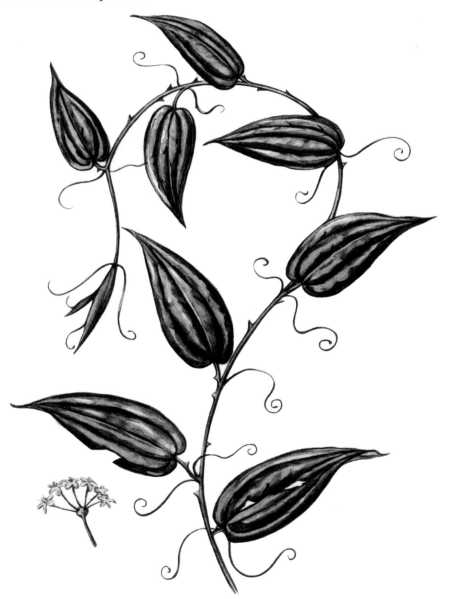

Indian sarsaparilla is a tonic, expectorant and aphrodisiac. It is renowned for clearing inflammation from the genito-urinary tract.

Description

Indian sarsaparilla is a slender plant with woody stems that climb or trail on the ground. Its vines grow from a tuberous, long-shaped root covered with dark brown bark that is cracked and contains fissures. The leaves range in shape from ovate to long and thin, and its small flowers are greenish-yellow on the outside and purple on the inside. Indian sarsaparilla grows throughout India, some of the Indonesian islands and Sri Lanka. An American sarsaparilla (*Smilax officinalis*) grows in the tropical areas of Central and South America.

Historical or mythological background

Sarsaparilla has been used as a medicine since ancient times, being regarded as an excellent protector of the liver. It has also been successfully employed in Ayurvedic medicine in the treatment of venereal diseases, such as syphilis. The ancient Chinese also valued sarsaparilla to treat syphilis. *Smilax officinalis*, the American sarsaparilla (a popular soft drink in the United States for many decades), was also used by the Native Americans as a tonic.

Modern uses

The roots of Indian sarsaparilla are prized for their curative powers in male reproductive disorders. Syphilis, herpes and genital sores are some of the conditions effectively treated with sarsaparilla. Impotence and seminal weakness are reduced with support from sarsaparilla's aphrodisiac

Indian sarsaparilla balances blood, vata and pitta; cures vomiting, pyrexia and bleeding disorders along with improving absorption.
—Raja Vallabha Nighantu
[An ancient Ayurvedic text]

effect. It is also applied externally and taken internally for skin conditions such as leprosy and psoriasis and is a traditional remedy for conjunctivitis. As a nervine tonic, it is given for neuralgia, epilepsy and psychiatric disturbances.

Available forms

Indian sarsaparilla dried root and whole herb is generally available from Chinese and Ayurvedic herb suppliers. Classical Ayurvedic combinations containing Indian sarsaparilla are usually labeled by their Sanskrit name—sariba. A famous traditional formulation is the herbal wine Saribadyasava, a blood purifier for

rheumatism and syphilis. A fortifying sarsaparilla drink made in a syrupy palm-sugar base called sharbath is available in India.

Home remedies

A traditional Ayurvedic blood-purifying remedy especially useful in alleviating conditions of internal bleeding, piles, rashes or excessive pitta conditions is known as sonithamrutham kashayam. It contains equal parts of haritaki powder, Indian sarsaparilla root and neem-bark powder. Combine 1/3 cup of each of these three herbs to make one cup. Add this to 16 cups water. Boil for 1 minute, then simmer uncovered until the liquid is reduced to 4 cups. Strain well and drink 1 cup three times a day 30 minutes before meals.

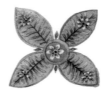

Senna (also known as Cassia)

Cassia angustifolia, East Indian senna, "King of the Trees,"
Tinnevelly senna
Sanskrit: Aragwadha *Hindi*: Sanay
FAMILY: Caesalpiniaceae

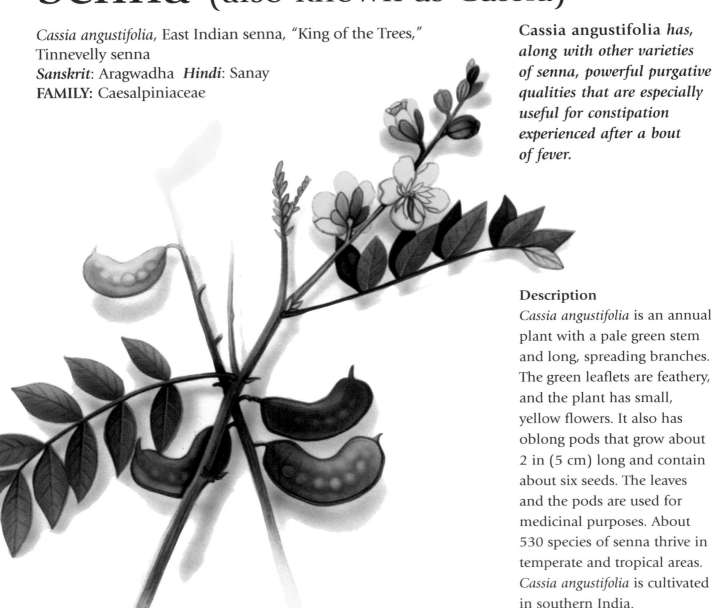

**Cassia angustifolia *has,
along with other varieties
of senna, powerful purgative
qualities that are especially
useful for constipation
experienced after a bout
of fever.***

Description
Cassia angustifolia is an annual
plant with a pale green stem
and long, spreading branches.
The green leaflets are feathery,
and the plant has small,
yellow flowers. It also has
oblong pods that grow about
2 in (5 cm) long and contain
about six seeds. The leaves
and the pods are used for
medicinal purposes. About
530 species of senna thrive in
temperate and tropical areas.
Cassia angustifolia is cultivated
in southern India.

> *Senna cures constipation, indigestion and disorders of the liver and spleen such as anemia, hepatitis and various forms of typhoid. It balances vata and kapha.*
> Ayurveda Vijnana
> *[An ancient Ayurvedic text]*

Historical or mythological background

Senna has been used for many centuries as a laxative. In the 9th century AD, upon the command of the caliph of Baghdad, two famous Arabian physicians found a safe laxative. They preferred the senna pods to the leaves; the ancient Greeks also used the pods. Senna was cultivated in England in the second half of the 17th century.

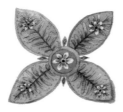

Modern uses

One of the safest herbal laxatives, senna helps to expel toxins, heat and acidity from the body. Senna also purifies the liver and spleen in conditions such as jaundice, spleen enlargement and fever. Pitta-predominant skin conditions, including leprosy and eczema, are commonly treated with senna in Ayurveda. Pure senna powder is virtually tasteless and can be taken with warm water before bed for constipation. Traditionally, senna is also used to rid the body of worms and to reduce flatulence. To reduce the griping that senna can cause, it can be mixed with asafetida and ginger.

Available forms

Senna powder, the most effective form of laxative, is obtainable from health food stores and herbal dispensaries. Its taste is quite bland, and since its effect is drying, it must be taken with plenty of warm water. Senna tea bags and tablets are also sold in health food stores and selected pharmacies.

Home remedies

To use senna as a laxative, take 1 heaped tsp in 1 cup ginger tea. You can replace the tea with warm water, but the ginger reduces the senna's possible cramping effect. Alternatively, you can take a senna tea bag in a cup of hot water. To boost the digestive cleansing effect, senna is given with equal parts of triphala before bed. Taking this after a fast helps to regulate the bowels again while flushing out deeper toxins.

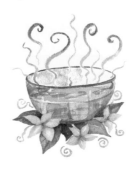

Shatavari

Asparagus racemosus, Women's treasure, Sparrowgrass
Sanskrit: Shatavari *Hindi:* Shatavar, Satamuli
FAMILY: Liliaceae

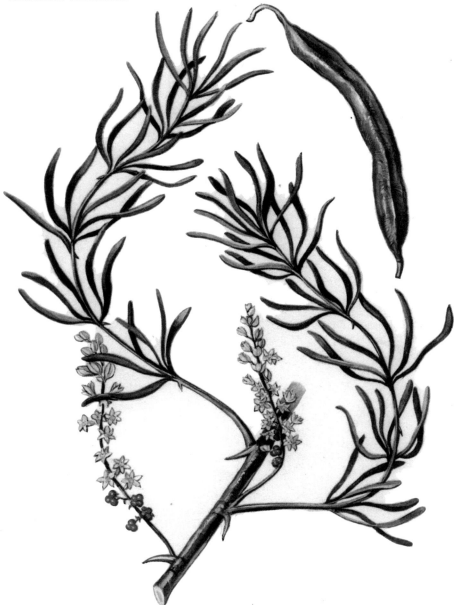

Shatavari is renowned as an excellent rejuvenative tonic for women and as a brain tonic that prevents fatigue.

Description

Shatavari is a climbing plant with many branches, a tuberous root, small leaves, white flowers and berries that are dark purple when ripe. The roots are about 12–36 in (30–100 cm) in length. The roots are used for medicinal purposes. The plant is grown and cultivated throughout India, growing well up to 4,200 ft (1,400 m) above sea level.

Historical or mythological background

Known as "a woman with a hundred husbands," shatavari (a form of asparagus) has been traditionally used in Ayurvedic medicine as a fertility tonic for women. The herb was renowned for increasing sexual libido and for treating impotence and frigidity. In

China, wild asparagus root (*Asparagus lucidus*) would be chewed to help alleviate symptoms of infertility. The Chinese believed that the root was capable of promoting compassion and an openness to feeling truly loved.

Modern uses

As the reigning queen of female reproductive tonics, shatavari is also known as "having the strength to satisfy 100 husbands." A strongly alkalizing and demulcent herb, shatavari is very soothing for acidic or inflamed mucous membranes that accompany sore throats, urinary tract infections, ulcers, bronchitis and kidney infections. Shatavari's ability to increase milk, semen and ovum production is indicative of its hormone-promoting capacity. As such, it is Ayurveda's primary fertility tonic. Shatavari's pitta-balancing effect can be applied to treat menopausal hot flashes and vaginal dryness. Research suggests it may play a future role in the treatment of serious disorders, including malignant tumors, lung abscesses and tuberculosis.

Available forms

Shatavari is often prescribed in the form of a powder, ghee or jam. The plant is hardy and easy to grow in warm climates. Traditional Ayurvedic formulations include shatavari gulam, a female reproductive jam, and shatavari mandura, a combination of shatavari and dairy products for painful periods and infant colic.

Home remedies

To enhance the function of the female reproductive system, especially in the treatment of menstrual irregularity and infertility or to regularize the reproductive system after a miscarriage, take 1 tsp shatavari powder in a cup of warm, unhomogenized milk before bed. For irritable bowel syndrome, combine:
1 part shatavari powder,
2 parts arrowroot powder
plus 2 parts musta (nut grass) powder. Take ¾ tsp of this compound in ½ cup warm water three times daily between meals.

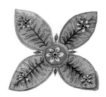

Shatavari is cooling, bitter and sweet in taste. It is excellent in healing disorders of the blood and for balancing vata and pitta conditions. One of the best tonics for female fertility and a powerful rejuvenator, it improves the memory and brain function.
—Dhanwantari Nighantu
[An ancient Ayurvedic text]

Turmeric

Curcuma longa
Sanskrit: Haridra *Hindi:* Haldi
FAMILY: Zingiberaceae

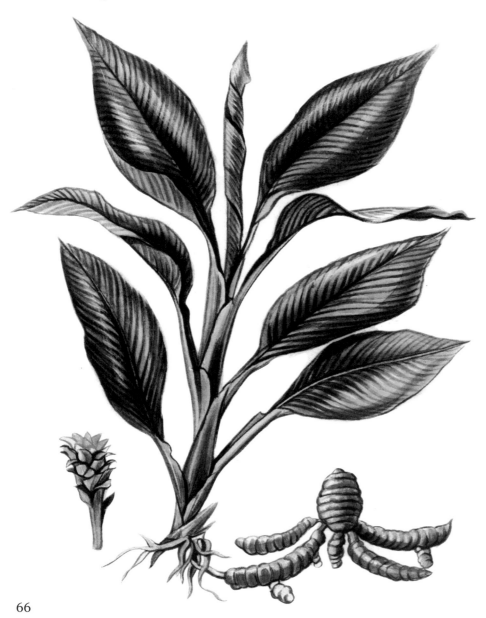

Turmeric is a natural antibiotic and an excellent stimulant for the metabolism. It is also a digestive and a blood purifier.

Description

Turmeric is a perennial plant that has tuberous, oblong roots, long, narrow root leaves, and yellow flowers that grow on top of the long central stem rising from the root. The pulpy root, which is yellow on the outside and orange–red on the inside, is used for medicinal purposes. The root, measuring up to 2 ft (60 cm) long, has also been used for dyeing food and fabric since ancient times, as it can function as a cheap substitute for saffron. In medieval Europe, turmeric was known as Indian saffron. Turmeric is grown throughout India and Southern Asia and cultivated in China and Java.

Historical or mythological background

In India, turmeric is symbolic of the Divine Mother and is believed to be able to attract prosperity. It has been used as an effective rich yellow dye. Brides are ritually bathed with turmeric before marriage to purify their body and to give their skin a glowing hue. Turmeric aids the practitioners of yoga by helping the flexibility of the ligaments and by clearing psychic blockages along the chakras. Yoga philosophy teaches that the body has seven chakras or energy centers situated vertically up the body, close to the position of the spine.

Modern uses

Turmeric is an antiseptic, antioxidant and antibiotic herb that every kitchen should stock. Sprinkled into almost every Indian curry and bean dish, its blood-purifying and bile-stimulating properties assist the digestive organs to assimilate food without forming toxic byproducts. It specifically boosts liver and pancreatic function, which is relevant to the treatment of diabetes, hepatitis, liver tumors and jaundice. Turmeric can also be applied to wounds, ulcers, boils, pimples or bites to prevent infection and to accelerate healing.

Available forms

The strongest form of turmeric is the fresh root, which can be grated and added to food or made into an infusion. This can be found in Indian and Asian grocery stores. The next best option is the powder, which can be purchased from most grocery stores and taken with plenty of warm water. Be careful when preparing turmeric, as it will stain anything it touches.

Home remedies

Turmeric combines well with neem and aloe vera to purify the blood and liver, particularly in conditions of pitta excess, such as after eating highly spiced and heated foods. Combine $\frac{1}{2}$ tsp ground turmeric, $\frac{1}{2}$ tsp neem leaf powder, 20 ml aloe vera juice. Mix the above combination well, consuming it twice daily, at mid-morning and before bed. Turmeric's natural antiseptic properties also make it an effective gargle. Add to 1 cup boiled water, $\frac{1}{2}$ tsp sea or rock salt, $\frac{1}{2}$ tsp turmeric and 3 drops tea tree essential oil. Gargle for a few minutes three to four times a day.

> *Turmeric balances kapha and pitta; cures dermatitis, anemia, edema, copious urination and ulcers.*
> —Raja Vallabha Nighantu
> *[An ancient Ayurvedic text]*

Winter Cherry (Indian ginseng)

Withania somnifera
Sanskrit: Ashwagandha **Hindi:** Asgandh, Punir
FAMILY: Solanaceae

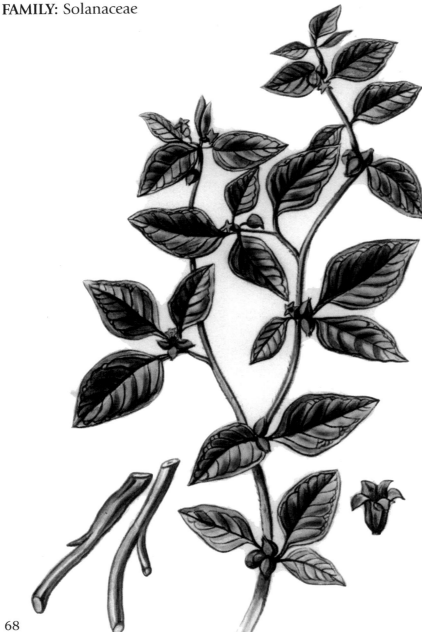

Winter cherry is a tonic, stimulant and aphrodisiac. It is renowned for helping alleviate insomnia and nervous tension.

Description

Indian ginseng is a perennial evergreen plant that grows from a fleshy, tapered root. The shrub grows to 4–5 ft (1.2–1.5 m) high. It has medium-sized ovate leaves, green or yellow flowers and globular, orange berries.
The root is covered with a light-brown thin bark. Inside the root, the juicy fibers are white. Indian ginseng grows wild in dry wasteland and is also cultivated for medicinal purposes. *Panax schin-seng*, or Chinese ginseng, is also used in Ayurvedic medicine. This type of ginseng is native to eastern Asia and is cultivated in Korea and Japan.

Historical or mythological background

Winter cherry, used in India for at least 5,000 years, was also known to Greek physicians such as Theophrastus. Winter cherry is also referred to as "Indian ginseng" because its properties were similar to the ginseng used in Chinese medicine. Chinese-cultivated ginseng has been used medicinally in China and Tibet since 3000 BC. In China, the roots were called Jin-chen, meaning like a man, referring to the shape of the root. Both Chinese ginseng and winter cherry can be combined to create a tonic to enhance rejuvenation for the patient.

Modern uses

Winter cherry is a fortifying remedy to counter modern stresses by strengthening the adrenals, which are usually depleted by stress. This accelerates recovery from nervous exhaustion and general fatigue. Winter cherry lowers blood pressure and sedates the nervous system. This is useful for hyperactive but debilitated

people. The Sanskrit name for winter cherry, ashwagandha, literally means to be "as strong as a stallion," referring to its powerful aphrodisiac properties. Used to slow the aging process, it reduces graying and serum cholesterol, as well as stimulating memory regeneration.

Available forms

Winter cherry is available in many forms. In India and some Asian countries, it is prescribed in various traditional combinations, including an invigorating herbal wine called ashwagandharishtam and a fortifying jam known as *ashwagandadhi lehyam*. In Western countries, it is available as a raw herb, fluid

> Ashwagandha is pungent, bitter and warm in potency. It tones, cures vata diseases such as cough, dyspnea, depletion and chronic ulcers.
> —Raja Nighantu
> [An ancient Ayurvedic text]

extract, tablets, powder or tincture from herbalists and selected health food stores.

Home remedies

For a dynamic energy boost, mix equal parts Indian ginseng, Siberian ginseng, licorice root and brahmi with four times the amount of water. Bring to a boil, simmer for 10 minutes covered and leave to steep until cool enough to drink. One cup of this in the morning will keep your mind and body alert throughout the day. As a male reproductive rejuvenative, 5 grams winter cherry powder can be mixed with 1 cup warm, unhomogenized milk, 1 tsp honey, 2 strands saffron, $\frac{1}{4}$ tsp long pepper and $\frac{1}{2}$ tsp pure ghee. This can be taken before bed every night for one month before conception. A period of celibacy can also be observed during this time.

Healing through Ayurveda

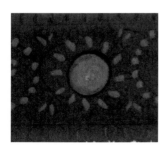

Ayurvedic View of Health & Disease

Ayurveda is a comprehensive, holistic system of healing based on the premise that health is our natural state of being, while disease is caused by an imbalance of the mind, body or soul. Ayurveda can be used to work out how to rebalance the body and mind to alleviate the symptoms of disease. Seeking health through harmony, Ayurveda can also be used as a guide to a balanced lifestyle that will maintain your health and extend your lifespan. Over five thousand years, Ayurvedic practitioners developed insights into healthy daily and seasonal maintenance routines, dietary regimes and therapies to alleviate any early signs of disease, as well as to enhance the health of the body and the stability of the mind.

It is traditionally believed that the basis of the Ayurvedic system stemmed from in-depth observations of nature. It was the *rishis* or sages that made these observations during extensive periods of meditation in natural surroundings in ancient India. They came to the conclusion that all things are connected and that we can find health if we follow the laws of nature. Our very existence is believed to be the combination of two great forces, one called Purusha (Great Spirit) and the other prakruti (Great Nature or Great Matter). Our connection with nature and

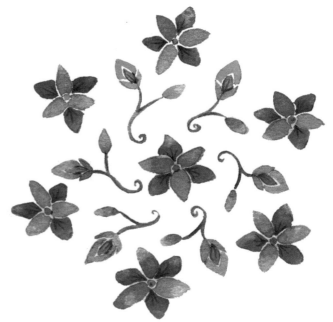

its wisdom means that if the laws of nature are followed, we find health, mental clarity and spiritual wisdom. If these laws are not followed, we encounter disease, mental confusion and separation from spiritual guidance.

According to those laws of nature, we are made up of a combination of the same elements that comprise the world and the cosmos—ether, air, fire, water and earth (see page 8). These elements (called bhutas) are also the five states of matter (prakruti)—ethereal, gaseous, radiant, liquid and solid—that combine to make up the three doshas (collectively called tridoshas) or body types—vata, pitta and kapha. To maintain a balanced dosha, Ayurvedic practitioners will recommend a food regime (see pages 81–87) or lifestyle changes (see pages 90–93) that are suitable for your particular body type.

There are also foods, therapies and strategies that are called tridoshic, which means that they help balance all doshas. Imbalances in the doshas can result from sudden shocks and traumas, or over time as a result of a stressful lifestyle, a poor diet, a buildup of toxins (ama) or poor digestive fire (agni). In Ayurveda, disease is called amayam, derived from the word ama, which is the buildup of toxins in the body. Each body type may manifest different kinds of imbalances that, if not checked, can develop into a serious disease. See the table below to identify the early and late stages of disease for the tridoshas.

Our minds are also a combination of three energies called gunas (collectively called trigunas) that make up our mental constitution—satva, rajas, and tamas. Each guna is also present in different types of food. Satva is a harmonious energy that corresponds with intelligence, calm and stability. In Ayurvedic medicine, satva is the desired emotional state of being for both health and emotional stability. Certain herbs, foods and lifestyles are satvic in nature and encourage a similar state in our bodies. Satvic energy is evident in herbs and berries used medically, such as holy basil and gooseberry, food that has been freshly picked and organically grown, and a calm, relaxed lifestyle. Satvic foods increase longevity, tranquility and spiritual awareness. Satvic people tend to be efficient in handling matters, are stable in their thinking and emotions, and do not tend to worry or get anxious.

PROGRESS OF DISEASE	EARLY INDICATIONS	LATE INDICATIONS
Vata	*Buildup of gas*	*Over-excitable mind and loss of memory* *Bloating and distension of stomach, shifting pains* *Feelings of insecurity, restlessness*
Pitta	*Buildup of heat*	*Excess anger and irritability* *Burning sensations, headaches* *Feelings of frustration, fear, hatred and jealousy*
Kapha	*Buildup of mucus*	*Cloudy thinking processes and lethargy* *Asthma, bronchitis, excess weight, water retention* *Obsessive behavior, depression*

The other two types of energy are useful in aiding energy imbalances but are not ideal states in themselves. Rajas energy corresponds to hyperactivity, passionate emotions and aggressive behavior. Rajasic foods, such as meat, hot spices, stimulants and intoxicants, increase mental agitation, anger, libido and hyperactivity. Rajasic people always feel dissatisfied with their lives, and are constantly searching for fame or more material acquisitions. Tamas energy corresponds to inactivity, apathy, and stagnation, and is increased by overcooked, stale, tinned or leftover food. Tamasic people tend to procrastinate and avoid work.

These types of energies, unlike the doshas or body types, are in a constant state of flux and, apart from satva, can indicate a state of mind that is inclined to particular types of imbalances. For instance, rajasic people may tend toward violent behavior, while tamasic people may suffer from addictive behavior.

This fundamental concept of the connection between the body, mind and spirit with the earth and cosmos makes Ayurvedic medicine and methods of approaching the prevention and cure of disease very effective. Used for over 5,000 years, and providing a basis for both ancient Chinese and Greek medicine, Ayurveda can be implemented to prevent disease (see pages 76–77), to purify the body of toxins (see pages 78–79) and to rejuvenate the system to increase longevity (see page 80). Body therapies (see pages 94–95) and beauty regimes (see pages 96–97s) can also be chosen according to your body type, as well as tridoshic therapies and regimes.

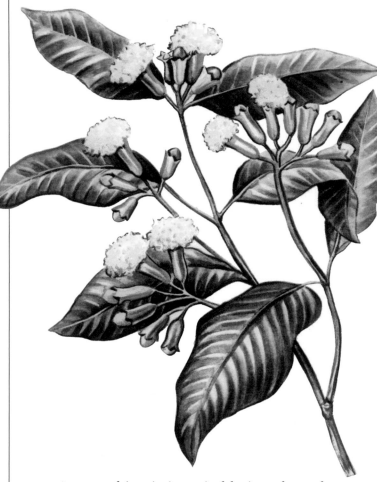

As everything is inextricably interdependent, all the things we do, experience, eat and feel have repercussions on our body, mind and soul. When treating illnesses, Ayurvedic physicians also take into account spiritual factors, such as the flow of energy through the *chakras*, the seven centers through which spiritual energy (called sushumna) runs. The chakras are positioned along the spine from its base to the top of the head. By focusing on spiritual balance, the effect on the spirit of physical and emotional disturbances can be alleviated. Clearing such energy blocks and feeling more focused and balanced as a preparation for a meditation can all be achieved by visualizing a flow of energy or life-breath through these energy centers.

The first chakra, located at the base of the spine, relates to feelings of security and sexuality, as well as to the reproductive organs, legs and feet, while the second chakra, positioned in the center of the pelvis, concerns setting emotional boundaries and corresponds to the spleen, ovaries, kidneys, urinary tract and the adrenals. The third chakra is located near the navel. Its energy is linked to willpower and self-image issues, as well as to the digestion, pancreas, liver, stomach, small intestines and blood sugar, while the fourth chakra, positioned at the heart, is linked to trust and flexibility. This chakra relates to the heart, the thymus gland, the lungs and the immune system. The fifth chakra is found at the throat, and its energy is related to communication, creativity and comprehension, as well as to the thyroid, neck, ears, sinus and throat. The sixth chakra is positioned in the middle of the forehead and relates to the intuition and the pituitary gland, the eyes and the nervous system. The seventh chakra is positioned at the top of the head, and its energy is directed toward enightenment, peace, Divine love and compassion. This chakra relates to the pineal gland, the hair and the central nervous system. In another system, there are nine chakra energy centers, with an extra chakra (called *Lalana*) positioned in the palate and the other (called *Manas*) slightly above the sixth chakra.

SAHASARA CHAKRA

The seventh chakra is positioned at the top of the head and corresponds to enlightment and peace.

AJNA CHAKRA

The sixth chakra, the "Third Eye," is located at the eyebrow center and brings intuition.

VISHUDDHA CHAKRA

Located at the base of the throat, this is the fifth energy center and relates to communication, creativity, and comprehension.

ANAHATA CHAKRA

The fourth chakra is positioned at the heart and is linked to trust and love.

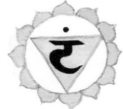

MANIPURA CHAKRA

The third chakra is located at the solar plexus. Its energy is linked to willpower and self-image.

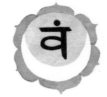

SWADHISHTANA CHAKRA

The second chakra is positioned in the center of the pelvis and concerns setting emotional boundaries. and reproduction.

MULADHARA CHAKRA

The first chakra is located at the base of the spine and relates to feelings of security, sexuality and social interaction.

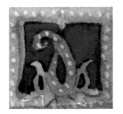

Preventative health

Strengthening the immune system and improving the digestion

Preventative health starts by strengthening the immune system. In Ayurvedic medicine, a kind of substance or sap called *ojas* is believed to protect the immune system from disease and the aura around your body from negativity and other destructive ethereal forces. Ojas is an essence resulting from the creation of the following seven types of tissues (called dhatus) of the body:

1. Plasma (rasa) nourishing the body.
2. Blood (rakta) energizing the body.
3. Muscle (mainsa) fleshing out the body.
4. Fat (meda) lubricating the body.
5. Bones (asthi) supporting the body.
6. Marrow (majja) filling the body.
7. Sexual fluids (shukra)—the source of the body's immunity and fertility; and ojas—the essence of immunity.

Except for the first type of tissue, each stage of development of the tissues in the body is dependent on the successful completion of the stage before it. The seventh stage of tissue production is called shukra, and it is from this stage that ojas is finally created. It is believed that the ojas can be stored in the body and that it should not be depleted. As shukra concerns procreation, excessive sexual activity will deplete ojas, as will sleeplessness, emotional trauma, poor diet and lack of exercise.

One of the diagnostic tools used by Ayurvedic practitioners is tongue diagnosis, in which such indications as the shape, thickness, texture, color and movement of the tongue are studied to reveal the condition of the body. A simple way of ascertaining whether your level of ojas is low involves sticking your tongue out. If it is shaking in this extended position, you may need to improve the integrity of your immune system. Other indications of low ojas include low levels of strength, lethargy, lack of interest and premature aging. Low ojas is also linked to Chronic Fatigue Syndrome (see pages 108–109).

Sweet-tasting herbs and satvic aphrodisiacs are believed to promote ojas. These sweet-tasting herbs include fennel, licorice and marshmallow, while Satvic aphrodisiacs include winter cherry, lotus seeds and shatavari. It is also believed that a sweet temperament will help increase ojas. In Ayurveda, important ways of improving your health include acting with kindness, honesty and compassion.

When the digestive fire (agni) is balanced (see also pages 7, 12–13), the nutrition derived from food is assimilated and directed toward keeping these seven types of tissues healthy, building up the levels of ojas in the body. A balanced digestion will also help in the efficacious elimination of waste products from the body. When the digestion is poor, the digestive fire (agni) is insufficient to transform the energy of the food into healthy tissue. The production of ojas suffers while the immune system is slowly undermined.

A number of straightforward indications of poor digestion exist, such as a poor appetite, indigestion, bloating of the stomach, lethargy and unrefreshing sleep. Poor digestion is also indicated by weight loss or weight gain. Check your tongue. Is it coated? Does it look or feel slightly swollen? If it is thickly coated or very furry, this is a sign that you have a buildup of toxins in your body. If the tongue is only mildly coated, this is an early warning that toxins are accumulating and that your store of energy is low. If your tongue has indents around the periphery, you are not utilizing your nutrients by absorbing them into the tissues. When they are not absorbed, the nutrients turn into waste products that are either poorly eliminated or stored in the body.

Overeating is one of the main causes of poor assimilation or digestion of food. Indigestion can be caused by long-term emotional stress; the suppression of your emotions, such as anger, grief and fear; or the failure to resolve these feelings. This type of stress can affect how your food is digested and can lead to an improper selection of food.

Another aid to digestion is eating foods that are beneficial to your dosha or body type and avoiding those that are detrimental for you (see pages 81–87). In Ayurveda, it is believed that there are three pillars of health—nutrition, harmony in relationships and rejuvenation. Concerning the proper intake of food, there is a list of foods that all doshas must avoid, which includes cold foods and drinks, as well as leftovers.

To improve your digestion, Ayurvedic practitioners recommend several strategies that should be observed before, during and after eating. Before eating, it is important to assess whether you are actually hungry. Hunger is an indication that a previous meal has been digested. It usually takes approximately five hours before a meal is completely digested. Also, try to eat in a positive state of mind, in pleasant surroundings and with good company. Never initiate an argument during meal times.

Do not eat your meal in a rush; chew each mouthful at least ten to twenty times, really savoring the taste. Sometimes we bolt our food down with little appreciation of its flavor. Once you have taken the time to enjoy your food, you may find that you start refining what you would really like to eat rather than just eating what is convenient.

In Ayurveda, it is important to limit your intake of liquids with a meal, as this can dilute the digestive fire in your stomach. If your digestion is weak or if you are a kapha type, take a warm drink before a meal. There is a rule of thirds in Ayurvedic medicine concerning the intake of food and drink. The rule states that you should fill a third of your stomach with food, another third with liquid, with the final third left empty to aid digestion. Once you have finished your meal, take a half-hour break to clean up and enjoy a short, slow-paced walk. Avoid the temptation to fall asleep after a meal, as this may produce toxins.

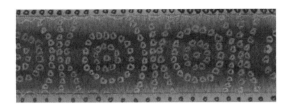

Purification therapies

Purification therapies aim to remove toxins that have built up in the body due to improper digestion. These toxins (ama) are basically undigested food particles, and, like mucus, they are heavy, cold and wet in quality. They slow down digestion and are the root of all disease (see also page 7). Ama is particularly responsible for most types of colds and fevers and autoimmune conditions. The principal objective of Ayurvedic purification or detoxification therapies is the elimination of the ama from the body. Only then can a person seek to implement a healthier lifestyle and food regime, and to undertake rejuvenation strategies. Different doshas or body types manifest ama in the following ways:

- Vata—distended stomach and bloating after meals, foul smelling breath, gray coating on the tongue, constipation and a poor appetite;
- Pitta—heavy feeling in the stomach after food, bitter taste in the mouth, yellow coating on the tongue, yellow stools and no appetite, diarrhea;
- Kapha—general feeling of pain and fatigue in the body, sour or salty taste in the mouth, congested chest and a poor appetite.

These conditions are called *sama* (with ama). The aim is to transform the body's sama condition to a nirama or normal condition. Generally, bitter or pungent herbs tend to be useful in breaking down ama. Bitter herbs include aloe vera, dandelion and echinacea, while pungent herbs include holy basil, black pepper, cardamom, cinnamon, coriander, cumin, garlic and ginger. Sweet, salty or sour-tasting food should be reduced during the detoxification process.

As each dosha manifests ama in different ways, slightly different techniques are used for each to purify the body. For vata types, ama is best removed by the use of digestive herbs in cooking and, in the case of trikatu, taken in supplement form after each meal. The body's metabolism should be stimulated by the use of carminative herbs, such as asafetida and cumin, for a short period of time. Only when the body is stimulated and the ama has been loosened can vata types use laxatives, such as castor oil, to clear the released toxins from the body.

For pitta types, purification includes the use of bitter- and sweet-tasting herbs, as well as bitter tonics. As pitta types are prone to overheating and fevers when unwell, bitter tonics (such as aloe vera juice and neem) are used in Ayurvedic medicine to disperse the inappropriate heat from the body. For kapha types, ama purification requires strong remedies because this type already naturally has a tendency to accumulate ama in the system. This body type requires both pungent- and astringent-tasting herbs, such as ginger, turmeric and long pepper.

Suggested two-week routine

A simple way of helping purify the body is to implement the following strategies for two weeks:

- *Drink a cup of warm water with ¹/₂ teaspoon triphala powder;*
- *Drink 20 ml aloe vera juice before bed; and*
- *Eat a light, vegetarian diet, using herbs suitable for your body type in your cooking and use only small amounts of salt.*

To assist in weight loss, drink half a cup of warm water or herbal tea once every waking hour.

If you have access to an Ayurvedic clinic or practitioner, you can choose to undergo a thorough purification process called *panchakarma*. This series of treatments effectively removes a buildup of ama by the use of such strategies as laxatives to flush ama from the intestines, as well as oil massage and steam to remove toxins from the skin. Again, panchakarma is devised according to your body type. However, before undergoing panchakarma, there are a number of things you need to change so that once the toxins are removed, you won't allow them to accumulate again.

This preliminary stage (called purvakarma) in the purification procedure requires you to change your eating patterns so that you are eating foods that are lightly spiced and are pacifying to your body type rather than aggravating to it (see pages 81–87). About ten other therapies can also be used to remove toxins, including steam therapy, and the use of herbal tonics and oil massages. Oil massages can be self-administered (see pages 94–95) or given by a professional practitioner.

To help with the purification process, Ayurveda also prescribes the eating of certain foods (see pages 81–87 for a listing of foods and tastes for the tridoshas), the wearing of garments of certain colors, a particular lifestyle regime and the recommended meditations to engage in. See pages 90–93 for further information about balancing lifestyles for your body type.

Some purification strategies for the tridoshas

VATA TYPES—short fasts of 1–2 days; wearing warm colors and white; meditations focused on quietening the mind; silence and burning sandalwood, frankincense incense or essential oils;

PITTA TYPES—fasts of up to 3–4 days; wearing cool colors and white; meditations focused on love and acceptance; avoiding heat and burning rose and sandalwood incense or essential oils;

KAPHA TYPE—fasts of up to a week; wearing warm colors; walking meditations and chanting; and burning sage, frankincense and myrrh incense or essential oils.

Long fasts are not encouraged in Ayurveda, especially for vata types, although kapha types are able to do fasts of up to a week without stressing the metabolism. If you have never fasted before, seek the advice of an Ayurvedic practitioner or other health-care professional.

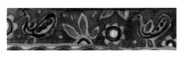 Longevity strategies

To enhance longevity, Ayurvedic medicine developed a range of strategies to help rejuvenate the body. In Ayurveda, special rasayana (rejuvenation) herbs combined with a diet to balance your body type (see pages 88–89), as well as a routine and lifestyle that complements your body type (see pages 90–93), are believed to lead to a better quality of life and to prevent the onset of serious diseases. The word rasayana is derived from the word rasa, which is the first type of tissue (relating to plasma nourishing the body—see page 76). If nutrients from the foods suitable for your body type do not infiltrate this first level of tissue metabolism, the ability of these nutrients to continue nourishing the six other levels of tissue types is greatly diminished.

In Ayurvedic medicine, old age is believed to be an autoimmune problem, which is linked to the depletion of the ojas that should be stored in the body (see page 76–77). It is also believed that by lowering the body's temperature and decreasing food intake to a healthy minimum, a person may live longer. The need for strict control of the diet is strongly advocated, with a predominance of sweet tastes, such as the taking of grains, honey, ghee and milk. These foods are believed to be the most effective foods for rejuvenation purposes. A number of rejuvenating herbs are found in Ayurvedic medicine, such as brahmi (see pages 22–23), gooseberry (see pages 42–43), shatavari (see pages 64–65) and winter cherry (see pages 68–69). For a list of rejuvenative foods, see page 89.

In Ayurveda, herbs are categorized according to their effect on the seven tissue types. Rejuvenation tonics (called rasayana karma) are those that nourish specific tissues, being calming to the nerves along with harmonizing the body and mind. Those herbs used for rejuvenation have a high quality of their own plant-like ojas, which imbues the plant with the ability to improve our tissue longevity, as well as promote clear thinking, a sense of joyfulness and physical health.

Ayurvedic rejuvenation therapies also include taking a retreat from the world to rest the senses and to give yourself time in which to release emotional toxins, such as fear, as well as to rebalance yourself. Retreats for up to a month are advised for those seeking to rejuvenate their lives. These retreats are believed to be most effective when you can avoid human contact (other than your physician) for the entire period of the retreat.

Simple rejuvenation ideas

- Take plenty of herbal teas, and vegetable and fruit juices suitable for your body type.
- Take a one-day, silent retreat each week when you can be by yourself to meditate and commune with nature.
- Choose to fast for one day each week, generally making sure that it is the same day each week and a day when you can rest, for instance on Sunday.
- Meditate for fifteen minutes each day.

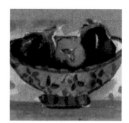

Food regimes

Even food, which is the life of all living beings, if taken in an improper manner destroys life.
While poison, which is by nature destructive of life, if taken in a proper manner acts as an elixir.
Charaka Samhita—*ancient Ayurvedic text*

Ayurvedic food regimes are chosen according to your body type. Each body type has its own tendencies toward imbalance, and, in Ayurveda, food is one of the most important ways of correcting that imbalance. A particular body type can aim to have a diet with the types of food that are compatible with that body type. As with herbs, foods, such as vegetables, fruits, grains and oils, can be categorized as vata-, pitta- or kapha-pacifying foods. If you choose foods that are pacifying to your body type, you give your body a chance to rest and to rebalance. An imbalance in your body type can manifest in a number of different ways, such as:

- If you are a vata type—food imbalances may mean that you feel extremely nervous and perform erratically at work or behave that way in your relationships.

- If you are a pitta type—food imbalances may mean that you feel angry, frustrated and overworked, and act in a domineering fashion in your relationships.

- If you are a kapha type—food imbalances may mean that you feel lethargic and slow, that you do not meet deadlines or finish your work, or that you tend toward co-dependent relationships.

In Ayurveda, it is believed that your food affects not only your body, but your mind and emotions as well. When preparing and cooking your food, it is important that you are in a harmonious mood. When you are eating, always choose pleasant surroundings in which to have your meal. If you are eating alone, make sure that you focus on your food and concentrate on the various tastes on your plate. Having the six tastes—sweet, sour, salty, pungent, bitter and astringent—represented in one meal is believed to be beneficial. Ayurvedic food strategies tend toward vegetarianism, identifying meat as having a tamasic and rajasic effect on the mind, emotions and body (see pages 71–72).

The following description outlines the food regimes for the different body types. The Ayurvedic system is also aligned with eating according to the seasons. This particularly affects those with dual body types. If you are a combined vata/pitta or pitta/vata type, follow the vata food regime during fall and winter and the pitta food regime during spring and summer. For dual pitta/kapha or kapha/pitta types, follow the pitta food regime during summer and early autumn and the kapha diet for the rest of the year.

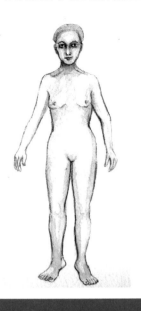

Vata

One of the best ways to ground and pacify a vata constitution is to eat your meals at regular times, with special emphasis on having a solid breakfast. Start your day with a hot glass of water laced with a few thin slices of ginger root. Prepare a warm breakfast of oatmeal or stewed fruits seasoned with some warming spices, like cinnamon and nutmeg. Choose flat bread, sourdough bread or any bread without yeast. You may have a warm drink after the meal, if your digestion is strong enough. Choose a herbal tea, such as chamomile or cinnamon, or warm, unhomogenized

FAVORABLE FOODS

INCLUDE SWEET, SOUR OR SALTY FOODS IN YOUR DIET

**VEGETABLES
(cooked only)**
Asparagus
Beets
Carrots
Green beans
Leeks
Pumpkin
Squash
Sweet potato

FRUIT (generally sweet)
Apricot
Banana
Dates, Figs
Grapes
Grapefruit
Lemon
Mango
Orange

Peach
Pineapple
Raspberries, Strawberries

GRAINS (well cooked)
Oats, Quinoa, Rice

BEANS (well cooked)
Split mung beans

**DAIRY (most dairy
tolerated in moderation)**
Ghee, Milk, Sour cream
Yogurt

**NUTS AND SEEDS (most
tolerated in moderation)**
Almonds, Cashews
Pumpkin and Sunflower
seeds

HERBS AND SPICES
Asafetida

Basil
Cardamom
Coriander
Cumin
Dill
Fennel
Garlic (cooked)
Mint
Mustard seed
Parsley
Peppermint

OILS
Almond
Corn
Ghee
Margarine
Olive
Sesame
Sunflower

SWEETENERS
Barley malt
Maple syrup
Brown rice syrup

TEAS
Bancha, Chamomile
Cinnamon, Clove
Fennel, Ginger
Lemongrass, Rosehip
Licorice

DRINKS
Almond milk
Aloe vera juice
Apricot juice
Carrot juice
Grain coffee
Grapefruit, Lemon, Lime
Pineapple juice
Miso broth

cow's milk with some spices, like cardamom, nutmeg or powdered ginger and a teaspoon of ghee. Consider having a spiced milk drink just before going to bed, to help you feel calmer and to promote a proper night's sleep.

For lunch or dinner, have some basmati or brown rice, which can be cooked with a teaspoon of oil, sea salt and some warming spices, such as mustard and cumin seeds. Combine the rice with cooked vegetables, such as zucchini, carrots, asparagus and green beans, or vegetarian curries featuring vegetables suitable for the vata body type. Avoid broccoli, cabbage, tomatoes and white potatoes. You can tolerate, in small amounts, lentils and mung beans, as well as spiced tofu.

FOODS TO AVOID

AVOID BITTER, PUNGENT OR ASTRINGENT FOODS, AND RAW FRUIT AND VEGETABLES

VEGETABLES (avoid frozen or dried vegetables)
Artichoke
Bean sprouts
Bell pepper
Broccoli
Brussels sprouts
Cabbage
Cauliflower
Eggplant
Endive
Leafy greens
Lettuce
Mushrooms
White potato
Tomato
Zucchini

FRUIT (avoid dried fruit)
Apple (red)
Cranberry
Pear (unripe)
Guava

GRAINS (avoid cereals)
Amaranth
Buckwheat
Corn
Millet
Oatbran
Rye

BEANS (avoid most beans)
Tempeh
Tofu

HERBS AND SPICES (avoid bitter and astringent tasting herbs and spices)
Allspice
Celery
Garlic (raw)
Horseradish
Marjoram
Nutmeg
Oregano
Paprika
Rosemary
Sage
Thyme

OILS
Canola
Mixed-vegetable oil
Peanut oil
Soy bean oil

SWEETENERS
Sugar substitutes
White sugar

TEAS
Alfalfa
Barley
Blackberry
Dandelion
Hibiscus
Orange pekoe

DRINKS (avoid alcohol and caffeine, carbonated, cold and chocolate drinks)
Apple juice
Berry juice (sour)
Cranberry juice
Coffee (decaffeinated)
Mixed vegetable juice
Pear juice
Soy milk

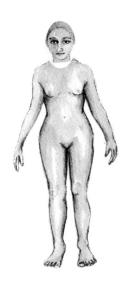

Pitta

Although pitta body types have the strongest digestive power, they should eat in moderation and choose to eat in a cool, shady, natural environment, ideally near a fountain. They should resist the temptation to eat their meals at their worktable. Upon waking, they should have a glass of water (at room temperature) with a couple of freshly picked mint leaves. Breakfast can consist of oatmeal sweetened with a few cardamom pods, powdered ginger, raisins and brown rice syrup or maple syrup.

Pitta types can usually tolerate wheat products. If you are not wheat sensitive, you could have a whole grain muffin or bread. High protein

FAVORABLE FOODS

INCLUDE SWEET, BITTER OR ASTRINGENT FOODS IN YOUR DIET

VEGETABLES (sweet and bitter)
Asparagus
Beans, Bean sprouts
Cabbage
Capsicum
Cauliflower
Celery
Cucumber
Eggplant
Leafy greens, Parsley
Peas
Pumpkin
Sweet potatoes
Zucchini

FRUITS (sweet)
Apple, Apricots, Banana
Cranberries, Dates, Figs

Grapes (sweet), Kiwifruit
Lime, Mango, Peaches
Pineapple, Pomegranate
Raisins, Watermelon

GRAINS (well cooked)
Barley, Couscous
Oatbran, Oats
Pasta, Rice, Wheat

BEANS (well-cooked)
Chickpeas, Kidney beans
Split mung beans
Pinto beans
Tofu

DAIRY
Butter (unsalted)
Buttermilk
Cheese (soft or unsalted)
Milk, Sour cream

NUTS AND SEEDS
Almonds (blanched)
Cashews
Pumpkin, Sunflower seeds

HERBS AND SPICES
Cardamom, Cinnamon
Cloves, Coriander
Dill, Mint, Nutmeg
Turmeric

OILS
Canola, Ghee, Olive
Soy, Sunflower

SWEETENERS
Maple syrup
Brown rice syrup
Sucanat

TEA
Bancha, Barley
Blackberry
Chamomile, Chicory
Cinnamon, Clove
Dandelion, Fennel
Hibiscus, Peppermint
Raspberry, Red clover
Spearmint

DRINKS
Apple
Almond drink
Aloe vera juice
Grain coffee
Grapefruit
Orange, Pineapple
Prune or Pomegranate juice
Rice and soy milk (boiled)

is favored by pitta types and can be included in a breakfast as scrambled tofu with a couple of cooling spices, such as coriander, cumin and saffron. It is best if pitta types cut down their salt intake and restrict themselves to sea salt or natural salt substitutes. For lunch and dinner, pitta types can eat light dairy products, such as cottage cheese. Pitta types should fill out their diet with a lot of lightly steamed or raw vegetables, bitter salad greens, certain fruits, such as apples and mangoes, basmati or brown rice and beans (except lentils).

Pitta types may drink during the meal; however, if suffering from indigestion, they should drink beverages before the meal. Beverages suitable for pitta types include bancha tea, barley-based drinks, fennel, licorice, lotus and marshmallow, and hot milk prepared with maple syrup and up to a teaspoon of coriander powder.

FOODS TO AVOID

AVOID SOUR, SALTY OR PUNGENT FOODS, AND ALCOHOL

VEGETABLES (avoid frozen, raw or dried vegetables)
Carrots
Chilies
Corn
Horseradish
Hot chili pepper
Leeks (raw)
Mushrooms
Onion
Pepper
Spinach
Tomatoes

FRUITS (avoid sour fruits)
Grapefruit
Lemon
Papaya
Strawberries

DAIRY
Butter (salted)
Cheese (hard)
Buttermilk (sour)
Yogurt

NUTS AND SEEDS
Brazil nuts
Hazelnuts
Macadamias
Peanuts
Pecans
Pinenuts
Pistachios
Walnuts

HERBS AND SPICES
Allspice, Asafetida
Basil, Bay leaf
Chili powder, Cloves
Fenugreek
Garlic, Ginger
Lemon thyme
Mustard seeds
Rosemary
Sage, Salt

OILS
Almond, Corn, Linseed
Margarine, Mustard
Safflower, Sesame

SWEETENERS
Honey, Molasses

TEAS
Basil
Cinnamon
Ginger
Ginseng
Juniper
Rosehip
Sage

DRINKS (avoid alcohol, coffee, carbonated and chocolate drinks)
Berry juice (sour)
Carrot juice
Lemonade
Miso broth
Tomato juice

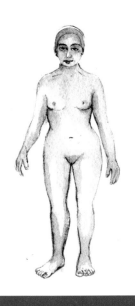

Kapha

Kapha body types need variety in their eating habits, and do best with a light, low-fat diet. For some, a dairy-free and wheat-free diet can be balancing. Upon waking, kapha types can have a hot glass of water with 1 teaspoon fresh lemon juice.

It is best for kapha types to drink their beverages before a meal. Beverages suitable for this body type include cinnamon, clove, orange peel, lemongrass or hibiscus-based herbal teas, or a fresh juice of carrot and ginger. Although this body type should limit dairy intake, drinking warm goat's milk with honey and a ¼ teaspoon of powdered ginger can still be beneficial.

FAVORABLE FOODS

INCLUDE BITTER, PUNGENT OR ASTRINGENT FOODS IN YOUR DIET

VEGETABLES (bitter and pungent)
Artichoke, Asparagus
Broccoli, Brussels sprouts
Cabbage, Carrot
Cauliflower, Corn
Garlic, Green beans
Horseradish, Leafy greens
Onions, Parsley
Peas, Spinach

FRUITS (astringent, not sweet)
Apples (green)
Cranberries, Grapefruit
Papaya, Pears (unripe)
Persimmons, Plums
Pomegranate, Strawberries

GRAINS
Amaranth, Barley
Basmati rice
Buckwheat
Cereal (puffed), Corn
Couscous, Millet, Oat bran
Oats (dry)
Polenta, Quinoa, Rye

BEANS
Adzuki beans
Black beans, Black-eyed beans, Broad beans, Chick peas, Lentils, Lima beans
Miso, Split mung beans
Peas

DAIRY
Buttermilk

NUTS AND SEEDS (in moderation)
Pumpkin and Sunflower seeds

HERBS AND SPICES
Allspice, Asafetida
Basil, Bay leaf
Black pepper
Cardamom, Cinnamon
Clove, Coriander, Cumin
Fennel
Garlic (cooked), Ginger
Lemon thyme
Marjoram, Mustard seed,
Paprika, Pepper, Rosemary
Sage, Tarragon, Turmeric

OILS
Canola, Mustard, Sesame
Sunflower

SWEETENERS
Honey (raw)

TEAS
Alfalfa, Bancha, Barley
Basil, Chamomile
Chicory, Cinnamon
Clove, Dandelion, Fennel
Ginger, Lemongrass
Orange peel, Peppermint
Raspberry, Red clover
Sage, Spearmint
Strawberry

DRINKS
Aloe vera juice
Apple cider, Carob
Carrot juice
Grain coffee
Pomegranate juice
Papaya juice

For breakfast, kapha types can choose to have fresh fruit, or fruit, such as apples or pears, stewed with cinnamon. If craving for bread, this body type does well with the occasional slice of toasted whole wheat bread with sugar-free jam. Breakfast can be followed by a cup of herbal tea, spiced with ginger, cloves or cinnamon. For lunch and dinner, this body type thrives on light, crispy food, and can have easily digestible grains, such as basmati rice (with some black pepper), and heating grains, such as rye, millet and barley. The grains can be combined with a hot, spicy mix of vegetables such as asparagus, carrots, cauliflower, eggplant and onions that have been sautéed with heating herbs, including hot peppers, and a teaspoon of a light, heating oil, such as mustard oil. Kapha types are encouraged to eat high fiber beans, such as aduki beans. Of all body types, kapha types should avoid having regular desserts.

FOODS TO AVOID

AVOID SWEET, SOUR OR SALTY FOODS, AND ALCOHOL

VEGETABLES (avoid sweet and oily vegetables)
Avocado
Bean sprouts
Capsicum
Cucumber
Eggplant
Mushrooms
Olives
Potato (white and sweet)
Pumpkin
Squash
Tomato
Zucchini

FRUITS (avoid sweet and sour fruits)
Apricot, Banana, Coconut
Figs (fresh), Grapes
Kiwi fruit, Lemon, Lime

Mango, Orange, Peach
Pear (ripe)
Prunes, Raisins, Raspberries

GRAINS
Bread (yeasted)
Oats (cooked)
Pancakes
Pasta, Rice, Wheat

BEANS
Kidney beans
Soy beans
Tempeh
Tofu

DAIRY
Butter, Cheese
Cream, Cow's milk
Sour cream, Yogurt

**NUTS AND SEEDS
(avoid all nuts)**

HERBS AND SPICES
Caraway
Poppy seed
Salt
Sesame seed

OILS
Almond, Apricot, Avocado
Coconut, Corn
Margarine, Olive
Safflower, Soy
Walnut

SWEETENERS
Barley malt, Brown sugar
Honey (cooked)
Maple syrup
White sugar

TEAS
Comfrey, Licorice
Marshmallow, Rosehip

DRINKS (avoid alcohol, carbonated, caffeinated and chocolate drinks)
Apricot juice, Almond milk, Banana shake
Coconut milk, Cold drinks
Grape juice, Grapefruit juice, Lemon juice
Lemonade, Miso broth
Milk, Orange juice
Pineapple juice
Peach juice, Pear juice
Prune juice, Rice milk
Tomato juice
Soy milk (cold)

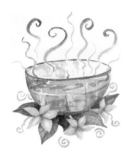

Medicinal foods

Without healthy food medicine is useless and with healthy food medicine is not needed.
Charaka Samhita—*ancient Ayurvedic text*

Healthy food is fuel for the body and ambrosia for the senses. Unhealthy or incompatible food feeds disease and promotes discomfort. As discussed above, food's physiological and psychological effects are based largely on the concept of the six tastes (rasas)—sweet, sour, salty, bitter, pungent and astringent. The tastes and their physical and mental effects, as well as the problems experienced in the body when a taste is taken in excess, are seen in the table below.

TASTE	EXAMPLE	PHYSICAL EFFECTS	MENTAL EFFECTS	EXCESS EFFECTS
Sweet	*Milk, rice, wheat, licorice, cane sugar*	*Nourishing, cooling, regenerates tissues, rejuvenative*	*Pacifies anger and fear, promotes contentment, attachment and love*	*Obesity, diabetes, swellings and lethargy*
Sour	*Rosehips, berries, lemon, tamarind, tomato*	*Stimulates digestive secretions and circulation, dispels gas, strengthening*	*Promotes mental awareness, stability and compassion*	*Blood impurities, muscle wasting, burning, anger and envy*
Salty	*Sea salt, seaweed, feta cheese*	*Enkindles digestive fire, laxative, demulcent, relieves contractions*	*Intensifies thoughts and emotions, fires inspiration, promotes courage*	*Vomiting, dehydration, kidney damage, water retention, bleeding, acidity, loss of hair/teeth*
Pungent	*Chilies, cloves, onion, garlic, mustard seed*	*Promotes digestion and secretions, purifies food, raises metabolism, stimulates circulation*	*Enhances passion, drive, alertness*	*Anger, nymphomania, emaciation, burning, dizziness and stabbing pains*
Bitter	*Aloe vera, bitter melon, turmeric, chicory*	*Sharpens taste, detoxifies blood and organs, anti-inflammatory, reduces fat and fever*	*Increases mental perception and focus loss, insecurity, grief*	*Emaciation, faintness, dehydration, memory*
Astringent	*Tannin tea, lentils, lotus seeds, guavas, plantain*	*Arrests bleeding, diarrhea and sweating, heals wounds, anti-inflammatory, raises prolapsed organs*	*Promotes memory and mental tranquility*	*Dehydration, constipation, skin pigmentation, heart pain, fear, confusion and dissatisfaction*

REJUVENATIVE FOODS

In Ayurvedic medicine, a number of foods can be taken regularly to promote health and longevity. These rejuvenative foods include the following:

Rice— Basmati is an aromatic rice with higher protein than white rice. Soupy rice is easily digested and strengthening during digestive upsets or convalescence.

Oats— High in calcium and inositol, oats soothe the nervous system and aid fat metabolism.

Asparagus— High in vitamin A and E, asparagus is a blood and kidney purifier.

Leafy green vegetables— A good source of antioxidant vitamins and minerals, these also purify the blood.

Apple— Reduces cholesterol and promotes healthy bowels.

Dates— A rejuvenative for the reproductive system and generally energizing.

Figs— High in iron and calcium, figs are a mild laxative and nutritive.

Mango— An invigorating fruit especially good for vata types in convalesence.

Grapefruit— Aids digestion of sugar and fat, along with liquifying mucus.

Split mung beans— Balancing for all doshas and highly nutritious, mung beans often form the basis for dahl.

Carob— An alkalizing chocolate substitute that has high calcium and protein.

Pure milk— Warm unhomogenized and unpasteurized milk strengthens the nervous system and enhances brain functions.

Almonds— A tonic for the kidney, brain, nerves, skin and reproductive system.

Sesame seeds— Rich in calcium and helps regulate the female reproductive system.

Olive oil— Containing the good HDL cholesterol, this oil is a liver and gallbladder tonic, as well as being nourishing for the hair and skin.

Ghee— Promotes memory, digestion, fertility, skin luster and tissue integrity.

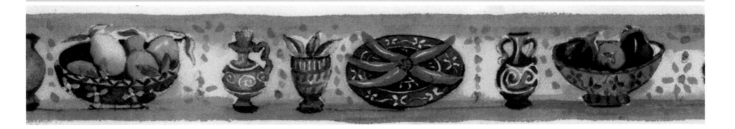

Lifestyle

One of the key features of a healthy lifestyle based on Ayurvedic principles is the adoption of a balanced routine of career, exercise and other lifestyle choices that pacify our predominant dosha or body type. This is in keeping with the Ayurvedic understanding that all things are connected, and that everything we do has an impact on our health.

On pages 92–93, we look at the ideal routine and lifestyle scenarios that help your body type stay balanced, allowing you to find health, stability and clarity. See if these lifestyles appeal to you, working out how closely they resemble your own lifestyle. Some may be surprised how their instincts have led them toward the path most beneficial to them. Others may find that they have been drawn to changing their lifestyle toward the Ayurvedic ideal, but have yet to implement it. At whichever stage you find yourself, it is important simply to work out how you would like your life to be, finding some guidance from the ancient wisdom of Ayurveda.

However, some lifestyle tips are relevant to all three doshas. As Ayurveda is based on the observation of nature, the three doshas are affected by the seasons. This means that at certain periods of the year, your body type will feel a little less balanced than at others. At these times, you must take particular care with your diet and ensure that you are observing at least some of the lifestyle choices that will help your body type to adapt to the changing seasons. Vata types usually find autumn slightly unbalancing as coldness and dryness causes dry skin and an increase in emotional upsets. Pitta types find summer particularly trying as the heat and sun cause skin rashes, internal heat, and anger. Kapha types need to take particular care during winter, when the coldness and wetness cause an increase in mucus, which can trigger colds and flus.

Some activities are considered good for all three body types, such as walking (the best time is between 6–10 am), working in the garden or tending your balcony plants, and practicing yoga. Yoga and Ayurveda have the same spiritual basis and are complementary systems. One exercise, called surya numaskara (or Salute to the Sun), balances and harmonizes all doshas. The exercise is believed to be a perfect balance between physical movement, clearing the mind and honoring of spirit. There are twelve postures, which should be performed in the morning, ideally at sunrise or sunset. Vata types should consider doing this exercise at the same time every day to encourage a feeling of routine in their lives. Pitta types will find that the exercise will help them feel calmer through the day, while kapha types will feel energized and encouraged to include more movement in their day.

HONORING THE SUN

1. *Stand straight with your legs and knees together and your hands in prayer position.*

2. *Inhale and stretch back your arms over your head as far as is comfortable.*

3. *Exhale and bend over, touching your toes. If you cannot reach your toes, try holding onto your shins.*

4. *Inhale and bend your knees and place your hands on either side of your feet, stretching the right foot back and placing your right knee on the floor. Arch your back and tilt your head back.*

5. *Retain your breath, stretch back your left foot and move your hips up into the "mountain" pose. Try to keep your heels on the floor.*

6. *Exhale as you lower your knees, chest and forehead down to the floor. Your hips should still be raised slightly higher than the rest of your body.*

7. *Inhale and lower your hips as you raise your upper body into the "cobra" position.*

8. *Exhale and raise your hips back into the mountain position.*

9. *Inhale and, leaving your hands where they are on the floor, bring your left foot forward, tucking the knee into your chest and keeping the right knee on the floor.*

10. *Exhale and straighten your left foot and bring your right foot forward, bending at the hips and keeping your hands on the floor or holding onto your shins.*

11. *Inhale and straighten your body, allowing your arms to sweep over your head and arching your spine back.*

12. *Exhale and return to standing with your feet together and your hands in prayer pose.*

Repeat the exercise, but this time change sides. Start with about one to three rounds on both sides and build up to ten or more rounds.

Caution: check with your health practitioner before commencing this exercise if you have a history of high blood pressure, heart-related problems or musculo–skeletal imbalances.

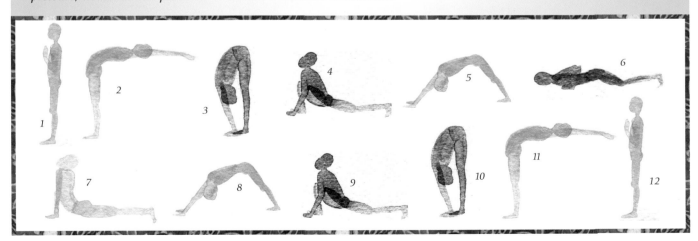

TRIDOSHIC ROUTINE FOR ALL BODY TYPES

The following routine lists all the various activities you may choose to adopt in your own daily practices, preferably in this order:

- *Awaken at sunrise;*
- *Close your eyes and "bathe" them with the light of the rising sun;*
- *Take five minutes to visualize yourself as healthy and happy;*
- *Brush your teeth and scrape your tongue (upon rising and retiring);*
- *Cleanse your nasal passages with warm, salty water (jala neti) or a therapeutic oil called anu thailam;*
- *Gargle with salty water or with water boiled with salt, basil leaf, and powdered ginger (do not drink this solution), and dry brush your skin with a natural bristle brush;*
- *Perform a self-massage (see page 94);*
- *Take a lukewarm bath or shower;*
- *Do the Salute to the Sun exercise (see page 91);*
- *Meditate for 15 minutes, choosing a meditation practice that suits you (see the purification strategies for all doshas on pages 78–79);*
- *Prepare each meal with care and visualize that the food is helping you become well or allowing you to maintain your health;*
- *Take a gentle, five-minute walk after each meal;*
- *Have a shower or bath after you have finished your day;*
- *Massage your feet;*
- *Meditate or listen to some soothing music; and*
- *Go to bed before 10 pm.*

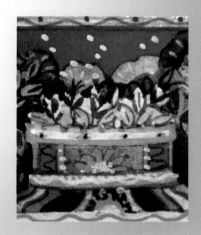

Vata

Vata types experience great fluctuations of energy, alternating between intense high energy and complete exhaustion. The only way to stop this unhealthy, reactive imbalance is to implement regulation. Routine is fundamentally important to vata types, and it includes eating at regular times. If you do not have a routine at the moment, consider implementing a regular regime until you have an adequate balance of work, rest and leisure time. Vata types must also consider introducing meditation into their life to help them feel grounded even if they are continuing their hectic pace of life. If self-employed, consider also taking a short nap during the afternoon.

Vata types should also concentrate on keeping warm and being in tranquil, moist, warm surroundings. Air-conditioning should be avoided, if possible, as the drying quality of the treated air aggravates vata imbalances. Jobs that will help vata types keep in balance include artistic endeavors in which their original thoughts can be best utilized, such as design, writing and acting. As vata types tend to search constantly for new experiences and fast-paced activities, it is advisable that they seek, during their leisure time, soothing and creative activities, such as painting or playing a musical instrument, which will help them calm down from the stresses of the day and quieten their overactive mind.

Pitta

Pitta types are usually very organized and practical in their approach to life, and are able to set and meet goals. They have a strong competitive streak that can make them seem intolerant of other people's shortcomings and find frustration and aggravation at work and even at play, if they choose competitive sports, such as tennis or squash. It is imperative that this body type works in cool, peaceful places, perhaps with a room fountain in their office. Because of their ability to organize their thoughts, delegate, and to bring their plans to fruition, they are often attracted to, and are suitable for, occupations such as lawyer, doctor, stockbroker, politician or company manager. However, if they are not careful, pitta types can become workaholics and distressingly difficult to work with.

To counterbalance pitta's overheated energies, they should consider choosing activities that are cooling and noncompetitive, such as swimming, or those that are done simply for the sake of enjoyment, such as a walking in the park. Avoid doing any exercise during the hottest part of the day and choose gentler leisure activities that can still exercise your active mind, such as chess. Also avoid wearing clothes that are tight-fitting and that contain synthetic fibers.

Kapha

Kapha body types tend to need a lot more stimulation and sheer physical activity during their day than the other two body types. Kapha types find routine easy to implement in their lives, making them excellent administrators, nurses and cooks. However, the routine may become so fixed for kapha types that they get stuck in a rut and find it difficult to change their procedures or routines.

When unbalanced, kapha types tend toward lethargy and inertia, sometimes needing to take a nap after their main meal. This body type needs to find the motivation to vary his or her routine—sometimes having a pet such as a dog can help kapha types go for long walks. They may choose to start a creative project to stimulate their senses or ensure that they have a lot of physical exercise both in their work and during their leisure time. Kapha types benefit particularly from hard physical labor or exercise, such as weightlifting, rowing and active team sports (like football or soccer). As kapha is the strongest body type of the three *doshas*, kapha types should generally aim to exercise to just before the point of strain, unless they are out of shape or suffering from a heart condition. This body type does best in a climate that is warm and dry.

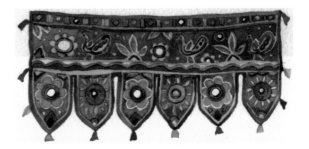

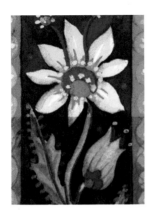

Body therapies
The art of self-massage

Daily self-massage promotes health, combats fatigue, strengthens the nervous system, improves eyesight, nourishes tissues, increases longevity, normalizes sleep, instills flexibility and strength as well as preventing and curing many diseases.
Vagbhata, Ayurvedic master

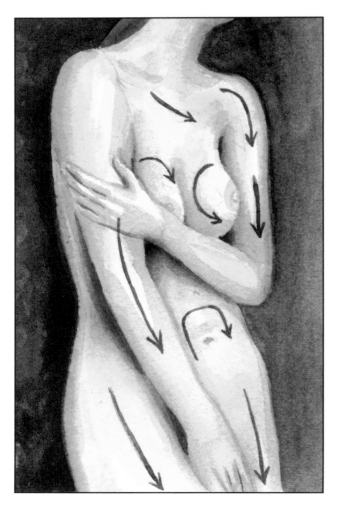

The sublime art of Ayurvedic body therapies has been developed and refined over 5,000 years. Massage is an integral part of Ayurveda and Indian culture, with children receiving massage from birth until they are seven years old. Among its countless benefits, massage improves circulation and elimination, strengthens the skin, hair, muscles and nerves and relaxes the mind. Self-massage cultivates a mood of self-awareness and nurturing that is essential for long-term health and happiness. It can be practiced at any time, but preferably at least 40 minutes before or after eating.

Vata types, who often suffer from dry skin and from being ungrounded, benefit from the moisturizing and grounding effect of massage. They respond well to warm sesame or castor oil with optional warming essential oils such as cinnamon, clove, geranium or sandalwood. Pitta types' propensity for inflamed skin is soothed by daily applications of coconut oil with cooling essential oils such as chamomile, lavender, jasmine or vetivert. Kapha types, with their predisposition for heaviness and accumulation, have to be careful not to use too much oil. If they have an accumulation of mucus, they should replace an oil massage with dry skin brushing using a natural soft bristle brush. Good oil combinations for kapha types include mustard oil or olive oil with cinnamon, ginger, frankincense, patchouli or sage.

The technique of self-massage is largely intuitive, employing a firm stroking motion along the bones, kneading fleshy areas and using circular motions around joints. Choose and warm the oil. Stand on a towel and start applying the oil to the entire body. Stroke the oil around each breast in a circular motion, then gently knead the shoulders. Follow with a long sculpting squeeze down the length of each arm. Massage the hands and around the finger joints. Then in the direction of the intestinal flow, massage the abdomen from the right hip, up the right side, across under the ribcage and down the left side.

With both hands, squeeze the oil down the thighs and calves following the direction of hair growth. You may like to sit down to comfortably massage the soles of the feet with your knuckles and stroke between the toes. Standing again, squeeze and knead the buttocks and stroke down the lower back with open palms. Massage the

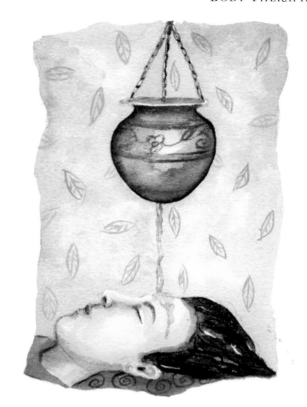

Shirodhara—a body therapy where herbal oil is poured continuously across the reclining patient's forehead.

back of the neck, the scalp and finish with your face. This oil can be left on for a minimum of 10 minutes and then washed off in the shower. The residual oil will leave your skin feeling soft and smooth.

OTHER SPECIALIZED AYURVEDIC BODY THERAPIES		
Body Therapy	*Method*	*Indication*
Shirodhara	*Herbal oil poured continuously across the reclining patient's forehead*	*Stress, hormonal imbalances, psychiatric problems, memory and hair loss*
Shirovasti	*Open-topped cap filled with oil as patient remains seated*	*Migraines, insomnia, tinnitis, epilepsy, cranial nerve problems*
Navarakizhi	*Herbal rice bolus dipped in herbal milk used for massage*	*Neuromuscular disorders, spine problems, osteoporosis*

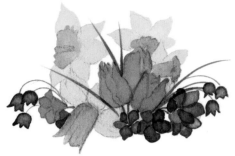

Beauty regimes

There is no cosmetic for beauty like happiness.
—Lady Blessington

Beyond the skin-deep effect of cosmetics, beauty is an inner radiance that is exuded from a person with a healthy body, balanced mind and loving spirit. Our outer appearance is a reflection of our inner state. When wastes are properly eliminated and nutrients are assimilated, this creates glowing skin, glossy hair, shining eyes, and strong hair and teeth. Ayurveda emphasizes the importance of a healthy diet, abundant fluids, regular sleep and exercise, massage, deep breathing and a relaxed, self-nurturing attitude.

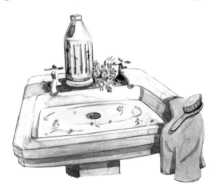

Drawing from nature's bounty, Ayurvedic beauty regimes feature fresh, edible products that are free from the possible risk of chemical allergic reactions associated with synthetic products. Since everything we put on our skin is absorbed into the bloodstream, a good rule of thumb is "if you can't eat it, don't feed it to your skin."

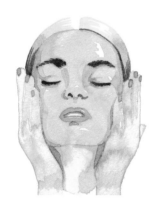

Cleansing Mask
Mix 12 parts chickpea flour, 1 part ground turmeric, 1 part sandalwood powder and 2 parts neem leaf powder. Add enough water to mix into a creamy paste. Apply to the face, neck and chest. Wash off after 10 minutes with a cloth dipped in cool water. Follow with a moisturizer or toner.

Moisturizing and exfoliating masks
The following ingredients for these masks, which vary for each body type, should be left on for 10 minutes:
- Vata—1 cup banana pulp and $\frac{1}{4}$ cup heavy (double) cream;
- Pitta—$\frac{1}{2}$ cup pineapple pulp, $\frac{1}{2}$ cup cucumber pulp and $\frac{1}{5}$ cup coconut milk; and
- Kapha—1 cup strawberry pulp.

Exfoliate

Mix 1 cup almond meal, 2 teaspoons ground cinnamon and 1/2 cup finely ground oats with enough water to make a creamy paste. Massage in a gentle circular motion, washing off after 2 minutes.

Body scrub

Mix together 1 cup Epsom salts, 1/2 cup chickpea flour, 1 tablespoon sandalwood or neem leaf powder, 1/2 teaspoon ground turmeric. Massage mixture over the body and wash it off after 2 minutes.

Toner

Combine equal parts rose water, witch hazel lotion, aloe vera juice and juiced cucumber. Place in atomizer in the fridge and spray on the face to rehydrate it.

Eyes

For clear bright eyes, apply Ayurvedic eyeliner (kajal) with camphor and castor oil daily. For bags or dark circles under eyes, combine 1 teaspoon of fennel seeds, 1 black tea bag, and 1 teaspoon of eyebright herb in 1 cup of water. Stir and allow to sit for 5 minutes. Strain and dip a cotton ball into the warm infusion, placing over your eyes and reclining for 5–10 minutes. This may be done daily.

Hair

Ayurvedic shampoos are so gentle on the hair that a conditioner is not required. Mix 2 cups pure coconut shampoo base or liquid olive soap base with 1 cup chickweed herb decoction and

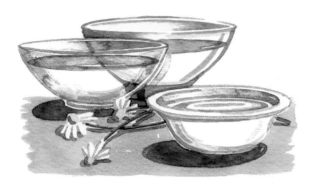

cup rosemary decoction. Add 10 drops of jasmine or sandalwood essential oil. To add lustre to your hair and cover any gray, rinse dark or red hair in henna powder and blonde hair in a strong chamomile infusion.

Scalp oil

For thick, glossy hair, use pure coconut oil massaged into the roots of your hair, or combine 1 cup gooseberry juice with 1 tablespoon licorice root and 1 teaspoon sandalwood powder. Add to 1 cup coconut oil and boil in an uncovered steel saucepan for 20 minutes. Strain and pour into a container. If you suffer from dandruff or psoriasis, add 2 teaspoons lime juice to each application. Massage the oil into the scalp every second day to prevent graying, hair loss and split ends, or once a week as a conditioning treatment.

Teeth

For healthy teeth and gums, massage them with warm sesame oil, strawberry pulp and a pinch of rock salt daily. For clean white teeth, floss daily and brush with a combination of aluminium-free baking soda, a pinch of neem leaf powder and a pinch of clove powder.

A-Z of Common Ailments

ACNE

Acne, a common problem among adolescents and young adults, is primarily a disorder of the oil glands in which the excess oil mixed with dead skin cells clogs the pores of the skin and generates small areas of infection. During adolescence, these oil glands may be unbalanced because of the high and unstable hormonal activity experienced during this period. Acne is often linked with symptoms of stress and a high-fat, high-salt and high-sugar diet.

Symptoms

Acne is the recurrent appearance of a number of pimples, blackheads and whiteheads on the face, upper back, shoulders, chest and upper arms. The most common form of acne is acne vulgaris. Severe cases of acne can take the form of cysts, which are infected swellings that form under the skin's surface. Rosacea, which is the frequent and sustained flushing of the face, creates acne-like symptoms on the cheeks and nose, because the pores of the skin are abnormally dilated.

Ayurvedic Treatment

Acne—whether cystic, teenage or rosacea—involves an increase in pitta or kapha. Sluggish elimination and poor liver function weakens the digestive fire, resulting in an accumulation of toxins (ama) in the bloodstream and the lymphatic system, which then overflows through the skin's pores. Externally, harsh, heating or chemical products should be avoided. Choose to use natural ingredients suitable for your body type (see pages 96–97). Internally, herbs can help to eliminate toxins, purify the blood and clear the lymphatic congestion. Some herbs to consider using regularly include turmeric, aloe vera juice, chlorophyll, picrorrhiza, manjistha, neem and triphala (a combination of gooseberry, bibhitaki and haritaki).

Lifestyle Changes

Foods that aggravate pitta and kapha tend to increase acne. To achieve and maintain a clear complexion, avoid excess oil, sugar, salt, chili, garlic, tomatoes, caffeine, citrus fruits, alcohol, nuts, red meat, yeast and dairy products. Favor a diet that is rich in natural chlorophyll, vitamins and minerals. This includes plenty of leafy green vegetables, ripe fruits, grains such as barley, pure water, seeds, and herbal teas such as fennel and chamomile. Try cooling sports such as swimming in fresh water or yoga. Daily self-massage will cultivate self-acceptance and improve the skin's texture and luster (see pages 94–95). Issues of low self-esteem and anxiety often underlie chronic acne. To uproot emotional causes, practice positive affirmations, visualizations and meditation.

Case Study

Sarah was a 23-year-old pitta constitution with cystic acne on her face and upper body. It worsened one week before her period and when under stress. Her diet included chocolate and a lot of orange juice. Exercise involved jogging at lunchtime under the noon sun. Sarah followed a pitta-reducing regime, which entailed cooling herbs, such as aloe vera juice, as well as primrose oil and shatavari powder to balance her hormones. She also eliminated heating foods, such as tomatoes, chocolate, citrus fruits, alcohol and red meat, from her diet. Instead of jogging, she took up yoga, which included cooling yogic breathing called *sheetali*. Psychologically, Sarah realized her acne acted as a "mask," which gave her an excuse to avoid social gatherings. Low self-esteem was gradually overcome by building a positive self-image through affirmations and visualizations.

ARTHRITIS

Arthritis, or inflammation of the joints, is believed to be a symptom of a dysfunctional immune system. Arthritis can also be caused by food allergies, which cause accumulated toxins. A number of joint diseases are known as arthritis, and there are two main types—osteoarthritis and rheumatoid arthritis.

Symptoms

Common in all forms of arthritis is pain in the joints. At first, this pain can occur intermittently, particularly when first getting out of bed or standing up. As the condition worsens, the pain can be felt during the night or in cold, damp conditions. Osteoarthritis, commonly experienced by the elderly, affects individual joints, such as the hips and knees. Rheumatoid arthritis affects the entire body, causing fatigue and anemia. In Ayurvedic medicine, the symptoms of arthritis are linked to imbalances of the three doshas or body types.

Ayurvedic Treatment

Treatment of arthritis varies according to the type suffered. Vata arthritis tends to strike suddenly with shifting sharp pains and accompanying cracking or popping of the joints. Pitta arthritis usually involves more burning, redness and nerve inflammation. Kapha arthritis improves with movement and is generally indicated by swelling and cold sensations. All types can often be linked to poor digestion and either a sedentary or an overactive lifestyle. A therapeutic approach includes digestive tonics such as triphala; anti-inflammatory Indian myrrh preparations; pain-killing antibacterials such as Indian frankincense; circulatory stimulants such as ginger and externally lubricating strengthening oils such as castor oil, mahanarayana oil, and punarnavadi oil to relieve the swelling.

Lifestyle Changes

A nutrition plan for arthritis is tailored according to the individual's doshic imbalance. For example, a person with pitta arthritis would be wise to follow a pitta diet. All doshas should avoid certain foods that can increase the inflammation and pain, such as sour foods, yogurt, tamarind, vinegar, pickles, citrus fruits, red meat and vegetables from the nightshade family (potatoes, tomatoes, eggplant and peppers). Sugar, cold foods and fried foods are also not recommended. Moving the joints every day through their full range will prevent the demineralization associated with osteoporosis and the settling of stagnant toxins associated with rheumatoid and nonrheumatoid arthritis. Specific yoga postures and symmetrical swimming or aqua-aerobics help to mobilize the toxins settled in the joints. Exposure to cold and damp weather should be minimized as it can often aggravate pain. Daily oil massage (see pages 94–95) and, in some cases, steam therapy may give relief.

Case Study

John suffered from malabsorption of nutrients for four years, and had started to experience pains in his finger joints during winter. He was advised to rub warm castor and ginger oil into his painful joints, as well as take a combination called mahayoggaraja guggulu, containing Indian myrrh. John had poor circulation, which improved with regular walking, self-massage and cinnamon/ginger tea. He was given an herbal combination of celery seed concentrate, Indian frankincense, long pepper and musta to stabilize digestive function. Reducing salt, alcohol, red meat and nightshade vegetables contributed to John's marked improvement after nine weeks.

ASTHMA

Asthma is a serious respiratory condition in which a series of factors, such as an infection of the lungs, emotional stress, physical distress and environmental factors (change in climate, air pollution, chemical fumes) can trigger an asthma attack. The causes of asthma are varied, and all aggravate an already sensitive immune system. The immune system itself may have been undermined by a number of factors, including adrenal exhaustion, low blood sugar and allergies to such airborne matter as dust, animal dander and mites. Allergies to certain foods may also contribute toward a vulnerable immune system.

Symptoms

One of the first signs of asthma is a feeling of restlessness and an inability to sleep, followed by tightness of the chest and a tendency to wheeze when breathing. Swelling in the bronchial tissues and a buildup of mucus narrow the lungs' airways. These symptoms are in response to an oversensitized response by the body to a presumed attack, which causes the need to cough in an attempt to alleviate the attendant congestion. As the condition worsens, other areas of the body experience tightness in the muscles, including the upper back and shoulders. In a full-blown asthma attack, a sense of suffocation is experienced with an increased inability to bring air into the body. As this occurs, the person experiencing the attack begins gulping for air, and is only able, because of panic and fear, to breathe into his or her upper chest, trapping stale air at the bottom of the lungs. Advanced attacks of asthma must be treated immediately as the symptoms can lead to fatality. When the attacks occur and how often they are experienced differ from person to person. Attacks can last from half an hour to several days.

Ayurvedic Treatment

Ayurveda traces the cause of asthma back to either an inherited respiratory weakness or acquired digestive inefficiency. Extreme fear and suppression of emotions are also related to the asthmatic condition. People with asthma tend to suffer from accumulated toxins in the stomach and accumulated phlegm in the chest. This sticky environment provides a fertile environment for allergens to take seed and can trigger a hypersensitive reaction in the mucous membranes, which results in an asthma attack. In order to prevent these incidents, the digestive and respiratory tracts must be cleansed and fortified. This is done by identifying and avoiding allergens, such as specific foods, dust, mold and pollens, until the body is strong enough to expel them before it overreacts to their presence. The body is then purified through treatments such as therapeutic vomiting, nasal cleansing and the use of herbs such as licorice, triphala, garlic, senna and long pepper. The specific herbs vary according to the individual's doshic imbalance. Strengthening breathing exercises (yogic pranayama) and herbal combinations are then given to promote dilation of the bronchial tubes and mucus expectoration, as well as building up the body's immunity so that the mucous membranes are no longer hypersensitive. Herbal combinations for this include trikatu (long pepper, pepper and ginger), sitopaladi churna (cinnamon, bamboo manna, long pepper, cardamon and rock sugar), and vasarishtam (with vasa and licorice). Herbal combinations to strengthen the immune system so as to prevent further asthma attacks include Ayurvedic jams—chyavanaprasham, agasthya rasayana, and kushmanda rasayana.

Lifestyle Changes

Regular aerobic exercise, such as swimming, is an effective way to manage asthma. Steam inhalation with essential oils of wintergreen, frankincense or rasnadi powder, followed by salt-water nasal cleansing (jala neti) and the application of a few drops of warm ghee up the nostrils can reduce the nasal passageway's hypersensitivity. Applying warm mustard seed oil or a camphor-based heating oil to the front and back of the chest daily can stimulate the dilation of the bronchial tubes and accelerate the expulsion of toxins. Supervised yogic-breathing exercises relax muscular and mental tension, thereby reducing the severity of attacks or preventing them altogether. Removing allergens from the home and diet until resistance has been built up is essential. Food allergies commonly associated with asthma include shellfish, mushrooms, peanuts, dairy products, meat, monosodium glutamate (MSG), cola, chocolate and wine. Allergens in the home include dust mites in carpets or curtains, mold in bathrooms and kitchens, and animal hair. Since colds often precede bronchial asthma, exposure to cold, damp weather should be avoided.

Case Study

Jasmine was an overweight 9-year-old with a kapha constitution who was experiencing breathlessness and asthma attacks every fortnight for 2 years. She was worse in winter and when she had a cold. Jasmine was put on a kapha-pacifying diet with particular emphasis on the reduction of dairy products, meat and oils. She started swimming bilateral breathing freestyle for 20 minutes daily and doing yogic breathing exercises. Since Jasmine was often constipated, she was advised to take a teaspoon of triphaladi powder daily (triphala plus licorice). A combination of equal parts trikatu and sitopaladi churna was also given three times daily. For acute attacks, Jasmine took a small dose of Euphorbia hirta and vasa, which effectively dilated the bronchial tubes. Within 5 months, Jasmine had gone off conventional medication; over the following 4 years, she only suffered, on average, one mild asthma attack a year.

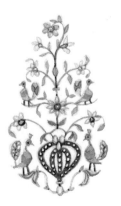

BOILS

Boils, also known as furuncles, are skin infections that occur in the pores of the skin, sometimes where there is a blocked hair follicle. They can appear on the face, neck and buttocks, and in the armpits. A boil appearing on the eyelid is called a sty.

Symptoms

A boil often starts as a red swelling. The bacteria of the infection mixes with the dead skin cells to create a swelling under the skin that grows as the white blood cells fill the area with pus. At this stage, a throbbing pain may manifest in the area. After about four to seven days, the boil usually bursts, letting the pus drain away and leaving the skin underneath clear of infection.

Ayurvedic Treatment

Boils are a sign of impure blood, poor immunity, excess heat and compromised liver function. Ayurveda resolves boils by prescribing a cooling and cleansing diet along with blood-purifying, antibacterial herbs. External poultices help to draw out the infection, reduce pain and promote scarless healing. Antibacterial herbs to cleanse the blood include neem leaf powder or decoction, aloe vera juice, Indian myrhh, sarsaparilla, turmeric, shatavari and triphala. Western echinacea and Swedish bitters are also excellent blood purifiers. A poultice of ground flaxseed soaked in a warm infusion of neem, sandalwood and turmeric is very effective for drawing out the pus, disinfecting the area and reducing inflammation.

Lifestyle Changes

Boils can easily spread and even multiply into painful carbuncle clusters if squeezed prematurely or if they are not disinfected regularly. Always disinfect clothes, bed sheets and other materials that have touched the boil. Keep the boil well coated in antiseptic cream such as neem seed oil, diluted tea tree oil or turmeric cream. The diet to reduce boils should suit the individual's doshic imbalance while pacifying pitta. Heating, fermenting and acidic foods such as yogurt, alcohol, red meat, tomatoes, chilies, onions, garlic, pickles, vinegar, yeast, sugar and sour fruits should be avoided. Coolants such as water, cucumber juice or fresh coconut water help flush out the impurities. Stay out of strong sun and avoid hot showers. Check blood sugar levels for underlying diabetes.

Case Study

Joshua was a 16-year-old pitta type with a boil under his right armpit. His blood sugar level was high and he overindulged in alcohol every weekend. Joshua took a combination of neem, turmeric, madhunashini, and fenugreek to stabilize his blood sugar levels. Daily doses of aloe vera juice and sarsaparilla were given to cool and purify the blood. A poultice of ground flaxseed, sandalwood, neem powder and turmeric was applied to draw out the infection. Once the head had burst, a comfrey ointment was applied to heal the area.

CANDIDA ALBICANS

Candida albicans is a yeast or fungus that lives in the bowel. A yeast infection occurs when the white blood cells in the bowel are exhausted through trauma, disease, or the use of antibiotics, which allows the yeast organisms to over-proliferate. As a result, women tend to experience vaginal infections, and as the condition worsens, toxins can be released to other moist environments of the body, such as the mouth.

Symptoms

Persistent, vague symptoms, such as tiredness, a coated tongue, flatulence, an itchy anus or vagina and fungal skin conditions can all indicate an over-proliferation of candida albicans. With vaginal infections, women may experience a swelling of the vulva and a thick, whitish discharge, while men may suffer red patches on the penis. Symptoms of oral thrush for babies include a white-coated tongue. Other symptoms include intestinal problems, such as gas, bloating, bowel irritation, constipation and diarrhea, and respiratory problems, such as throat and sinus infections, bronchitis and asthma.

Ayurvedic Treatment

Ayurveda sees candida as ama accumulation and takes a three-pronged approach—namely, to starve and kill the candida and to restore the healthy intestinal flora and the immune system. Antifungal herbs, such as neem, Indian myrrh, manjishta and triphala are highly effective in eliminating the candida fungus. Externally, antifungal herbs, such as neem oil and tea tree oil, are useful.

To alleviate the symptoms of vaginal thrush, dip an unbleached tampon in a mix of pure unsweetened yogurt and a little tea tree or neem oil. Insert the fresh medicated tampon every night for three consecutive nights. Western herbs such as pau d'arco, calendula and golden seal are also invaluable antifungal herbs. To support the remaining healthy flora and immune function, Ayurveda applies herbs such as Indian ginseng, garlic, shatavari, picrorrhiza and mineral bhasmas according to the individual's requirements.

Lifestyle Changes

Diet modification plays an essential role in the management of a candida albicans infection. Funguses or fermented foods should be temporarily withdrawn. These include alcohol, sugar, fruits, tempeh, mushrooms, soy sauce, cheese, yeast, honey, maple syrup, malt and caffeine. Nutrition can include plenty of high fiber, nutrient-rich foods such as vegetables, whole grains, culinary herbs and herbal teas. As candida is easily transmitted during sexual intercourse, condoms should be used to avoid infection. During menses, women suffering from a vaginal yeast infection should use pads instead of bleached tampons, as the tampons can trigger a reaction. Lactobacillus acidophilus yogurt or powder (at room temperature) should be taken daily. Avoid antibiotics and contraceptive pills, as they can easily aggravate the problem.

Case Study

Carmen was a 32-year-old vata constitution with a chronic case of candida albicans. Carmen was put on the anticandida diet and asked to drink lots of pau d'arco tea throughout the day. By applying calendula and neem oil externally, the itchiness around the groin subsided. Internally, she was given a combination of triphala, neem and asafetida to be taken twice daily. To strengthen the digestive and reproductive system, she was later put on a combination of shatavari and acidophilus until her energy was restored.

CHOLESTEROL PROBLEMS

The liver, intestines, fatty tissues and every cell in the body manufacture cholesterol. The body needs cholesterol for a number of reasons, including the production of certain hormones such as the sex and adrenal hormones, bile salts and vitamin D. One type of cholesterol, called high-density lipoprotein (HDL), returns excess cholesterol to the liver, where it is treated for elimination from the body, ensuring that a buildup of this type of cholesterol does not occur. This type of cholesterol is often referred to as "good" cholesterol. Low-density lipoprotein (LDL), or "bad" cholesterol, raises the level of cholesterol in the bloodstream by transporting the excess to the cells, resulting in the cholesterol remaining in the body.

Symptoms

The normal range of cholesterol is 180 mg/dl to 200 mg/dl. High cholesterol occurs when there is more than 200 mg/dl in the system. By itself it does not have recognizable symptoms, but it raises the risk of other diseases, such as heart disease, stroke, angina, high blood pressure and atherosclerosis (hardening of the arteries). Symptoms of these diseases include sharp pains and tightness in the chest, an irregular heartbeat that either flutters or pounds, difficulty breathing, fatigue and fluid retention in the ankles and legs. Studies have recently examined the effect on the brain cells when the body is low in cholesterol (less than 160 mg/dl). Low levels of cholesterol in the brain cells have affected access of these cells to an important chemical in the brain called serotonin. Serotonin is a neurotransmitter, a chemical produced from certain nutrients that effectively calms the mind, stabilizes the emotions and helps a person fall asleep. Where access is decreased, symptoms of sleeplessness, depression and anxiousness are often reported, as well as mood disturbances. The effect of low cholesterol on the body is only now being examined.

Ayurvedic Treatment

High cholesterol and pathologically low cholesterol are both considered health threats by Ayurveda. Since only 25 percent of our cholesterol comes from diet, understanding our own cholesterol production, emulsification, distribution and storage processes is an important concern. Research has shown that those with high levels of bad cholesterol (LDL) are more likely to be highly reactive to stress or to have poor liver or gall bladder function. The stress response triggers the release of hormones, such as adrenaline, which consist primarily of cholesterol. The more stress a person experiences, the more cholesterol the body has to make. Accordingly, stress management techniques are pivotal to lowering high cholesterol. When fat or cholesterol enters an ama-filled body, the cholesterol is more likely to clog the system and eventually become rancid (oxidize). Saturated fat from processed foods and cholesterol from animal products is more likely to elicit this rancid reaction. This may be why indigenous cultures with diets high in antioxidants— vitamin A, C, E, zinc—and bioflavonoids generally have a low incidence of cholesterol-related diseases. Ayurveda treats high cholesterol or low cholesterol by maximizing the digestion, giving a dosha-specific diet, teaching stress management with yoga or meditation, and supplementing the diet with herbs. Ayurveda's most effective tonics for high cholesterol are garlic, triphala guggulu, long pepper, vidanga, manjishta and punarnava. Those with extremely low cholesterol are advised to take ghee-based tonics such as ashwagandadhi lehyam.

Lifestyle Changes

Kapha people are more prone than the other body types to develop high cholesterol. This is because of their tendency to retain fat more so than vata and pitta body types. However, the driving ambition of pittas can create stress in their lives, elevating the body's cholesterol production. A diet low in cholesterol foods, including dairy products, meat, saturated fats, margarine, sunflower oil, caffeine, fried foods and alcohol, can help prevent cholesterol excess. Pittas would be wise to set aside unstructured time for leisure and meditation. They should also consider taking up an exercise program that is relaxing and noncompetitive. Foods that can keep LDL cholesterol levels low include oats, barley, corn, canola oil, flaxseed oil, olive oil, fruit juice (especially grape, grapefruit, apple and orange), millet, lecithin, quinoa, garlic, beans, almonds, walnuts, carrots, strawberries and other foods rich in vitamins A, C, E, carotenoids, and zinc. Smoking, alcohol, deep fried foods, saturated fats and red meat should be excluded from the diet.

Case Study

Norm was a 42-year-old journalist with high cholesterol. He smoked 8 cigarettes a day, drank 14 beers a week and rarely exercised. He was also unable to get an erection as his penis arteries were blocked with cholesterol. With the looming threat of heart disease acting as an impetus, Norm agreed to quit smoking, take up football and substitute the beers with 1 glass of wine daily. He also reduced his consumption of dairy products and red meat to twice weekly. After 3 months on a kapha-pacifying diet, Norm actually started to enjoy fresh juices, salads and hearty whole-grain cereals. Practicing a yogic relaxation technique called yoga nidra three times a week left him feeling much calmer. Yoga nidra is a perfect meditation for busy or mentally hyperactive people. It is a guided relaxation that lasts around 30 minutes, unwinding the mind and body. Tapes are available from most yoga centers or alternative bookstores. Taking an herbal formulation called triphala guggulu, along with a tincture of hawthorn berries (a cholesterol-lowering herb), returned Norm's cholesterol to a healthy level within four months. His ability to achieve an erection returned soon after.

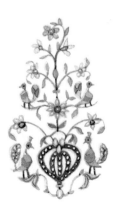

CHRONIC FATIGUE SYNDROME

Chronic Fatigue Syndrome (CFS) or Chronic Fatigue Immune Dysfunction Syndrome (CFIDS) is a debilitating condition that favors women under 45 years of age more than any other group. Sufferers of CFS experience an overwhelming fatigue that prevents them from carrying on many of the tasks of everyday living. Increased sleep does not bring relief from the condition. The onset of CFS can be sudden, with the intensity of the flu. Unlike the flu, CFS can last for at least six months, with the symptoms appearing, disappearing or shifting in intensity, apparently at random.

Symptoms

A large range of nonspecific symptoms can indicate Chronic Fatigue Syndrome in a patient. Symptoms go beyond merely feeling fatigued, and include chronic pain, loss of mental capacities, deep depression and digestive disturbances. Sufferers may also experience low-grade fever and a sore throat. However, unlike the common cold (see pages 112–113), CFS is fortunately neither contagious nor permanently debilitating. Other symptoms include insomnia or an inability to wake up easily in the morning, an inability to focus or concentrate and swollen lymph nodes.

Ayurvedic Treatment

Since Chronic Fatigue Syndrome constitutes a large range of nonspecific symptoms, treatment varies greatly from patient to patient. From an Ayurvedic perspective, CFS is due to depleted ojas, the sap-like substance that is connected with our immunity and vitality, which is produced from a balanced body and mind. The body is depleted because it is busy fighting an internal battle against undigested mental or physical toxins or unresolved infections. Without the energy reserves to expend on otherwise normal physiological or mental processes, a CFS sufferer is unable to cope with everyday challenges. As CFS is commonly related to a vata or kapha imbalance, general advice for balancing these body types is relevant. Initially, diet and herbs should be given to purify the organs and channels.

Purification practices known as panchakarma, involving treatments such as enemas or medicated vomiting, may be also appropriate (see pages 78–79). After panchakarma, herbs, gentle exercise and meditation may be used to rekindle the digestion, improve the immunity and nurture a positive attitude. To integrate this new, healthy pattern into the mind and body, rejuvenating body therapies, such as herbal oils and internal tonifying herbs, are used. It is important that the underlying toxic hotbed of ama has been eliminated before building up the body's strength and immunity. Failing to eliminate the ama will mean that any attempt to improve the immune system will be short-lived, as the toxins gradually wear down the body again.

Lifestyle Changes

In Ayurveda, disease results from the overuse, underuse or misuse of the body. This is particularly evident in CFS. Elite athletes, workaholics and perfectionists have a higher incidence of CFS due to the syndrome of overuse (ati-yoga). Without sufficient recuperation, the mind and body goes on strike, becoming unable to function at a satisfactory level. To reinstate equilibrium, a phase of inactivity may be required for a short time. By exploring new avenues for developing creativity, relationships and an inner serenity, CFS can become a blessing in disguise. It is also an indication that the time has come to be gentle and nurturing to the body rather than a thankless taskmaster. Self-massage, yoga nidra relaxation, meditation, cooking wholesome meals, connecting with nature and indulging in an enjoyable exercise or hobbies can all prove helpful. The diet should be as pure and as easy to digest as possible. Vegetable juices, steamed vegetables, soups, casseroles, digestive spices and whole grains suited to the body type are supportive to the cleansing and reparative process. Eliminate chemical-based products from the home and workplace and choose organic, additive-free foods, drinks, cleaning agents and paints.

Case Study

"We have won the right to be terminally exhausted."
Erica Jong, b. 1942

Gretchen was a 31-year-old mother of two with a vata constitution. She was also a nurse and a marathon runner. Gretchen contracted glandular fever, but continued her busy schedule until she finally broke down. Aching all over, feverish and bedridden for months, Gretchen felt her old active life slipping away. In a desperate effort for self-preservation, the body had enforced minimal activity. Gretchen underwent a purifying and strengthening panchakarma regime. In conjunction with daily massage and oil therapies, she took cleansing antiviral herbs such as cat's claw, long pepper, kantakari (*Solanum xanthocarpum*), guduchi and echinacea. A series of herbal oil enemas was followed by digestive herbs. Gentle qi-gong and walking were practiced daily. She adhered to the nutrition plan of fresh fruit, vegetables, whole-grains, digestive spices and culinary herbs, avoiding processed or preserved foods. After Gretchen's digestion returned to normal, the fever disappeared and her strength increased. Gretchen was prescribed adrenal tonic herbs including winter cherry, licorice and brahmi. After 5 months, Gretchen was able to return to life at a more modified, relaxed pace. To keep her immune system strong, she now takes chyavanaprash jam daily.

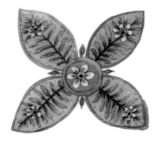

CIRCULATION (POOR)

Circulation problems occur when there are blockages or constrictions experienced in the blood-carrying passages, such as the arteries and veins. These blockages or constrictions may be caused by a number of factors, ranging from the serious consequences of the hardening of the arteries (which can lead to heart disease) and weakened arterial walls (which can lead to aneurysms) to the less threatening conditions caused by exposure to the cold (which can lead to chilblains), hemorrhoids and varicose veins.

Symptoms
While symptoms vary, a general sluggishness in the movement of blood and oxygen around the body can lead to a heightened sensitivity to cold in the peripheral parts of the body, or even memory loss. Other minor problems concerning poor circulation include chilblains, when the cold causes inflammation and pain to an exposed part of the body.

Ayurvedic Treatment
Vata and kapha body types have a greater tendency toward poor peripheral circulation than the pitta body type. Ginger, clove, gotu kola, cinnamon and brahmi are just some of the warm infusions that help fire the circulatory system. Adding pungent spices, such as ginger, pepper, cayenne, green chili and paprika, to your meals is another invaluable way to combat icy extremities. Sometimes vata body types also suffer from anemia and low blood pressure. In this case, tonics that are high in iron, such as red grapes, and cerebrovascular stimulants, such as brahmi and gingko biloba, are useful.

Lifestyle Changes
Warming your body with a daily self-massage is one of the best ways to optimize circulation. Vata body types can use warm sesame oil, kapha types—mustard oil, and pitta types—almond or jojoba oil. Adding a little cinnamon, juniper, rosemary or ginger essential oil to the base will increase its warming potency. Wearing warming colors, such as shades of red, brown, orange, yellow and black, can help to conserve body heat. Practicing half an hour of exercise daily promotes sweat and increases the heart rate and can also warm up the body. To prevent and treat varicose veins or spider veins, apply witch hazel lotion to the area while elevating the legs for 20 minutes daily.

Case Study
Shaemus was a 53-year-old with constantly cold hands and feet. He was also suffering from memory loss and hemorrhoids. Shaemus was asked to walk at a brisk pace, for 30 minutes daily. He also started to give himself a warm-oil massage for five minutes daily with sesame oil. In the evening, he had a bath with cinnamon essential oil. Daily intake of trikatu (black pepper, long pepper and ginger) started to improve his circulation within a week. A combination of brahmi and gingko biloba was later introduced to improve his memory. He also massaged his scalp with warm brahmi oil twice a week. Because hot spices may have aggravated his hemorrhoids, these were not added to his diet. External applications of witch hazel lotion on Shaemus's hemorrhoids helped them to shrink.

COLD SORES

Herpes simplex virus (type 1) causes cold sores, which are infections that occur mainly around the outside of the mouth, nose and fingers. There are a number of different types of the herpes virus—it is type 2 that causes sores around the genitalia. Cold sores are generally recurring once a person has contracted the virus, although many sufferers may build up their immunity so that they can defeat the virus completely. Cold sores can be contracted or flare up again during times of stress or when experiencing a fever or a lowering of immunity. Certain foods, which contain the amino acid arginine (such as chocolate), have also been linked to the flare-up of cold sores.

Symptoms
When cold sores first appear as blisters or inflamed sores, they are accompanied by fever, symptoms of the flu or swollen lymph nodes, with the initial, often mild, infections usually occurring during childhood. Recurrent episodes are usually free from these symptoms. Once the blister breaks, the area is covered with a yellowish crust, which drops off within 7 to 10 days.

Ayurvedic Treatment
Recurrent cold sores are a symptom of low immune function, a hypersensitive nervous system and unbalanced pitta or vata. To prevent an outbreak, protect the lips with an aloe vera, tea tree oil and vitamin E lip balm, reduce foods high in L-arginine (see next paragraph) and manage stress levels before becoming overwhelmed. Herbs to take to help clear the virus from the body include St. John's wort, neem, Indian myrhh, aloe vera juice, echinacea and kantakari (*Solanum xanthocarpum*). During an outbreak, cold ice on the area for 30 minutes can reduce severity. Apply a mixture of neem, aloe gel and ghee to accelerate healing.

Lifestyle Changes
Enjoy foods high in lysine and zinc, including brewers yeast, bean sprouts, fruits, vegetables, sunflower seeds and pumpkin seeds. Foods high in the amino acid L-arginine can exacerbate an attack, so should be avoided. These include chocolate, gelatine, chicken, wheat germ, peanuts, rye, corn, barley, soybeans, walnuts, cashews and carob. Regular meditation or guided relaxation can help to thwart an outbreak related to stress. Keep the immune system and nervous system strong with daily self-massage and herbs appropriate to the individual constitution. As herpes is highly contagious and can cause blindness if it affects the eyes, be careful to thoroughly disinfect hands or instruments that contact the area.

Case Study
Karen was a 24-year-old who suffered from herpes" outbreaks for the past year. She noticed they were worse during times of stress and when her nutrition was poor. Karen also suffered recurrent urinary tract infections, another sign of pitta imbalance. After following a pitta-reducing diet that was low in L-arginine and high in lysine, Karen found her outbreaks were less frequent. She also took triphala powder and aloe vera juice before bed to purify the blood and keep her immune system strong. Taking up mantra meditation, Karen was less vulnerable to stress and mood fluctuations.

COMMON COLD

Over two hundred viruses can cause you to feel cold symptoms. Attaching to the mucous membranes lining your nasal passages or throat, these viruses are first attacked by white blood cells known as neutrophils. However, these cells can work as an effective antibody only if they can exactly match the virus. The body is often unable to come up with the right antibody, as these viruses are constantly evolving and undergoing permutations. Known as an upper respiratory tract infection, colds are also believed to be the result of an immune system that has been undermined by such factors as inadequate rest, poor diet, and stress. These factors lead to a buildup of toxins in the body, so that the body's response to the intrusion of a viral infection is not effective as it has been busy coping with toxins arising internally. When the body's immune system is so lowered, it becomes prone to allergic reactions to certain foods and environmental triggers, such as dust and pollen. As the body becomes oversensitized, it is increasingly less able to withstand the onset of a virus.

Symptoms

Symptoms of a common cold appear about 2 days after infection. As soon as the body is aware of the infection, the neutrophils are sent to the infected area. This massing of the white blood cells causes the feeling of achiness in the area and is responsible for symptoms of inflammation. Colds may or may not be accompanied by a fever. Other symptoms, such as the increase of mucus in the nose and throat, fever, headaches, chest congestion, fatigue and loss of appetite, soon develop and will last from 1 to 4 days. The color of the mucus will often be light yellow in color. It is important to note that the first 3 days of a cold from the first sign of these symptoms are the

most contagious. The overall symptoms typically last for 3 to 4 days. Bronchitis, sinusitis and middle ear infections can occur as secondary infections. Bronchitis is characterized by an infection of the lungs' air passageways. Sufferers of bronchitis experience a slight fever and often a sore throat. The infection of, and build up of mucus in, the air passages constrict the progress of air to and from the lungs. If the inflammation worsens, the mucus becomes dark yellow in color and is often loosened by coughing. Where there are recurrent bouts of bronchitis, the condition may worsen into emphysema, causing the sufferer (who is usually elderly) to experience difficulty breathing out. Sinusitis is the inflammation of the sinus passages, usually those that surround the nose. Symptoms include nasal congestion, coughing, headaches and fatigue. A middle ear infection can accompany a common cold. Symptoms of middle ear infection include fever and an earache. Care must be taken not to blow the nose or cough too hard during the progress of a cold, as the infection in the throat can be pushed up into the ear.

Ayurvedic Treatment

The common cold is a classic example of how the body can undergo a progressive imbalance in all the doshas over a short time. The sequence of a cold begins with the body being exposed to stress, change, wind or cold. This creates a vata disturbance, which manifests as tiredness, restlessness, unusual pains, reduced appetite and loss of enthusiasm. Then the pitta phase sets in with fever, sweating and an irritated feeling in the throat, nose or eyes. As the cold progresses, kapha becomes dominant with copious mucus, lethargy and depression. At whatever stage a cold is, plenty of effective Ayurvedic home remedies are at hand. Holy basil is an excellent antibacterial, expectorant antiviral herb that can be used during all the phases. Cardamom, cinnamon, cloves, ginger and licorice help to warm the body and soothe the mucous membranes, while long pepper, pepper, ginger and lemongrass aid mucus expectoration. Turmeric, fenugreek and garlic help to purify the lymphatic system and dry up the mucus. Western herbalism offers boneset (*Eupatorium perfoliatum*) for the body ache, echinacea as an anti-viral and golden seal to strengthen mucous membranes.

Lifestyle Changes

Keeping warm and well rested is the best way to support inner healing powers to conquer a cold. The head, neck and feet are the most important areas to keep warm at all times. Frequent sips of warm tea with cinnamon, cloves, cardamom, holy basil, ginger and honey are usually very effective. Inhalation with tea tree, wintergreen, camphor or eucalyptus essential oil helps to liquify and expel the mucus while disinfecting the respiratory passageways. A nasal-cleansing yogic technique called jala neti assists in further flushing out nasal mucus. This involves pouring lukewarm, mildly salted water up one nostril and allowing it to flow out the other nostril. This is then repeated on the opposite nostril. It is best to see a demonstration by a yoga teacher or Ayurvedic practitioner before commencing this practise. Nasal drops of warm ghee, sesame oil or traditional *anu thailam* help to relieve vata sinusitis symptoms. Two drops in each nostril is generally sufficient. Rubbing warm mustard seed oil on the chest and back is an effective way to take the chill out of the body. A warm Epsom salts bath with heating essential oils such as ginger is also effective.

Case Study

Fleur kept getting a runny nose and achy muscles. She was given a diet to suit her kapha constitution, along with trikatu (long pepper, black pepper and dried ginger) and daily inhalation with wintergreen essential oil. Within a few days, she recovered from the cold. To prevent further recurrences Fleur took gooseberry powder daily for its vitamin C.

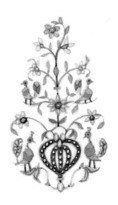

CONSTIPATION

Constipation occurs when the feces have dried in the colon and are difficult to pass from the system. This can occur for a number of reasons, including a poor diet with little fiber, a lack of adequate fluids and insufficient daily activity. Constipation can also occur if the urge to defecate has been repeatedly repressed. Other conditions such as pregnancy, irritable bowel syndrome, depression and an underactive thyroid can cause constipation.

Symptoms

Symptoms include difficulty passing the feces. As the feces stay in the colon for periods longer than three days, the body may experience abdominal bloating and an increase in gas. There has been great discussion about how often a person should defecate. In Ayurveda, the number of bowel movements a day should reflect the number of large meals you have eaten in a day.

Ayurvedic Treatment

Kaphas tend to get constipation due to lack of muscle tone and accumulation of toxins. Herbs that tone the intestine, such as triphala and dandelion, are suited for this, along with garlic, which contains an intestinal wall stimulant called allicin. Vatas' constipation is more likely to be triggered by dehydration, a change in routine such as when traveling, or stress. Lubricating laxatives such as flaxseed oil, castor oil or prune juice are very effective in remedying vata constipation. Although pittas are least likely to suffer constipation, when they do, it is often linked to inflammation or poor liver and gall bladder function. Cooling liver tonics, such as aloe vera juice, senna and dandelion, generally re-establish the elimination flow. Increasing fiber to bulk the intestine with psyllium husks is something from which all types may benefit.

Lifestyle Changes

The golden rules to bowel harmony can be summarized by the three f's: fluid, fiber and fitness. Plenty of warm fluids and liquid foods help to flush out undigested waste material. This is especially important during airplane flights, exercise, cold windy weather and hot temperatures. Conversely, dry, baked, fried or dehydrated foods in excess clog up the gastrointestinal tract. Mixing warm water with an adjunct such as chamomile helps it to absorb into the deeper tissues. Fiber stimulates the intestinal peristalsis involved in a bowel motion. Good sources of fiber include bran, fruits, vegetables, and whole grains. Fitness promotes healthy muscle tone and function, bringing toxins to the bowel and flushing them out. Excessive tension in the abdomen, however, can lead to a spastic colon, which disturbs elimination. To prevent this, one can squat and massage the abdomen in a clockwise direction.

Case Study

Emily was a 17-year-old vata constitution who had intermittent constipation all her life. She took a very low fiber diet and rarely drank more than 2 cups of tea a day. She was asked to eliminate white flour, white rice, dairy products and red meat from her diet. The bulk of Emily's meals now consist of brown rice, bean and vegetable casseroles with digestive spices and at least 6 cups of chamomile, licorice or fennel tea. Emily practiced a yogic colon cleanse called Shanka Prakshalana once a month for 4 months and took triphala. She now has a complete bowel motion daily.

COUGH/SORE THROAT

Coughs are the body's way of releasing mucus or irritants from the lungs, bronchioles and trachea. The reasons for coughing are various, such as to expel food swallowed the wrong way, to clear the lungs of mucus caused by infections in the upper airways, and to allay allergic reactions. Chronic sore throats can be caused by viruses, or may be due to lymphatic congestion causing infected tonsils.

Symptoms

There are three types of coughs—productive, nonproductive and reflex. When mucus is brought up, this type of cough is described as productive. Nonproductive coughs are dry coughs, such as those that can be caused by exposure to tobacco smoke. Reflex coughs occur as symptomatic of problems in other areas, such as acid reflux from the stomach. Sore throats are usually experienced as part of the common cold (see pages 112–113) and asthma (see pages 102–103). Other causes of sore throats include breathing through the mouth and infection by the streptococcal bacteria (strep throat).

Ayurvedic Treatment

Chronic sore throats can be due to lymphatic congestion causing infected tonsils. This can be treated by gargling with antibacterial combinations including tea tree, eucalyptus, golden seal, holy basil, cardamom, ginger, pepper, red sage, rock salt, turmeric, glycerine or honey. To cleanse the lymphatic system internally, fenugreek tea, garlic oil, thyme tincture and vasa are all excellent options. A dry, irritating cough may be due to an allergic reaction and can indicate the use of herbs that cleanse, soothe and strengthen the respiratory tract, such as coriander seeds and black cumin seeds. When the cough is productive of thick mucus, strong-acting herbs can be taken to prevent it from progressing to a serious infection. Such herbs include expectorants, such as ginger, long pepper and pepper, and antitussives that relax the bronchioles, such as vasa, licorice, holy basil, cumin, purified camphor, and palm sugar. To soothe the inflamed membranes, demulcent herbs such as marshmallow and warm milk with tumeric may be taken in the latter stages.

Lifestyle Changes

To preserve prana, vata types should keep talking to a minimum. Regulate airflow through gentle yogic breathing (pranayama) and steam inhalation with antibacterial essential oils such as tea tree. To reduce kapha, remove foods such as rice, dairy, and cold and raw foods from the menu. Heavy foods such as potatoes, bananas and red meat can be reduced. Plenty of warm herbal honeyed teas, such as a cinnamon, ginger, cardamom, clove, peppercorn and chai, help to dry up mucus and eliminate the underlying pathogen.

Case Study

Simon was a kapha constitution who suffered from coughs an average of twice yearly, which could cause bronchial asthma. He took sitopaladi churna powder, which consists of cinnamon, cardamom, long pepper, palm sugar and bamboo manna, as well as 3 cups of ginger, licorice, holy basil and honey tea a day. Once the mucus had loosened and bronchioles were opened, he underwent supervised yogic vomiting once a week for 6 weeks. This quickly expelled the accumulated mucus in the stomach, which was the origin of the problem. He later took trikatu (long pepper, ginger and black pepper) at any sign of sluggish digestion.

CUTS, STINGS, BITES

Shallow cuts made by a knife have clean edges and heal rapidly, while deep cuts can become infected, with a risk of scarring if the wound is spread open or not cleaned. Lacerations occur when the skin is cut by, among other things, broken glass, and the wound has jagged edges causing a greater risk of infection. Stings are categorized as those given by certain insects, spiders or marine life where the venom is injected into a person via the creature's stinger, whereas bites include those from such creatures as snakes.

Symptoms

Infection is the main concern for cuts, scratches and bites. Signs of infection include redness or swelling around the wound and discharges from the wound. Serious infection can result in fever and swollen lymph nodes. Long puncture wounds caused by long sharp objects, such as a rusty nail, may cause internal bleeding, and the person must be checked for tetanus. Depending on what caused a bite or sting, the symptoms vary, and include the affected area feeling sore or itchy or swollen. Sharp pains may be experienced in more serious cases, as well as fever, vomiting and difficult breathing.

Ayurvedic Treatment

A complete branch of Ayurveda called visha chikitsa specializes in the treatment of venomous bites and stings. However, here we will deal with less lethal bites and stings that can be safely treated at home. A traditional remedy to stop fresh cuts from bleeding and to promote healing is a paste of turmeric powder and honey. Dust the injured area with the powder and once the bleeding has ceased, apply a thin layer of honey. Organic honey such as manuka or tea tree has particularly strong antibacterial properties. This can then be covered with a sticking plaster or gauze. For stings or bites, apply the juice of coriander leaves and holy basil leaves. Neem seed oil can be applied to bites and stings later to keep infections at bay. Aloe vera gel and rosehip oil are excellent for promoting scarless healing in the resolution phase. A paste of ghee, honey, black sesame seeds and pure cow's urine is a traditional remedy to disinfect and reduce the pain of cuts, bites and stings.

Lifestyle Changes

To prevent bites, cuts or stings from getting infected, blood-purifying herbs such as aloe vera, neem, turmeric and manjishta can be taken internally. Neem is said to deter insects from biting or stinging when taken internally and applied externally. Once the damage has been done, substances to boost the immune system and promote healing are advised. Herbs with immuno-stimulant properties include gooseberries, shatavari, winter cherry and guduchi. To reduce itching, chickweed and shirisha are excellent herbs.

Case Study

Robert, a 12-year-old boy, cut his finger while playing with a pocketknife. After the wound was washed in diluted tea tree oil and hot water, it was dusted with a combination of turmeric and sandalwood powder. This was applied daily with a little ghee and was then covered by light gauze. After three days, aloe vera with rose hip oil was smoothed on the area twice daily to ensure that a scar did not form.

CYSTS (AND FIBROIDS) IN THE UTERUS

Cysts are swellings filled with fluid and dead skin cells that appear under the skin in many areas of the body, including the ovaries and the uterus. They are named after the area in which they are found. Ovarian cysts are common and, although in themselves harmless, may indicate in some women the presence of ovarian cancer. They generally only produce symptoms if they are interfering with some function of the organ to which they are attached, such as an ovarian cyst pressing on the bladder and causing frequent urination. Cystitis is a condition unrelated to cysts, being caused by bacteria traveling up from the urethra to the bladder. Fibroids are benign tumors that are attached to the walls of the uterus. They develop slowly and usually occur in women aged between 30 and 50.

Symptoms

Ovarian cysts often go undetected until they press on a neighboring organ, making sexual intercourse and ovulation painful, or twist and break (causing lower abdominal pain). Another common symptom is intermittent pain during menstruation. As fibroids tend to slowly continue growing, they become detected when they interfere with the menstrual flow, causing heavy or irregular bleeding accompanied by lower abdomen or lower back pain. Fibroids may also affect a woman's fertility or distort the shape of the uterus.

Ayurvedic Treatment

Growths such as ovarian cysts and uterine fibroids are indicative of a blockage of vata and a reflex accumulation of kapha and toxins in the bodily channels. To restore balance and proper elimination, Ayurveda initially ensures that the digestion is at optimal function. Then herbs are given to balance the body's hormone levels. A common combination prescribed is called sapthasaram kashayam. This is a mix of 7 herbs including ginger, castor root, bael roots and punarnava. It is very effective for dissolving and expelling growths. Warm castor oil poultices are also placed over the uterine region, along with daily self-massage.

Lifestyle Changes

In order to facilitate the purification process of menstruation, during the first three days, exercise should be kept to a minimum, sufficient sleep is advised, sex is to be avoided and pads are preferred to tampons in order to encourage an unobstructed flow. Heavy or oily foods, which increase estrogen synthesis in the body, are reduced. Restricted foods include meat and eggs. Sugar, salt, tea, coffee, soft drinks, fried foods, chocolate, cold foods and recreational drugs should be avoided. Daily self-massage and warm Epsom salts baths with clary sage essential oil are often helpful.

Case Study

Cassandra was a 35-year-old single woman with a history of two miscarriages. When investigating the cause, three large fibroids were discovered on the uterus. She was advised to go on a low-estrogen diet, and to use warm castor-oil packs on the lower abdomen daily. Given a combination of asafetida and saptasaram decoction, Cassandra's fibroids began to reduce after three months.

DEPRESSION

Many reasons can contribute to a person feeling depressed for prolonged periods of time. Bouts of depression may vary from several days to many years. Women occasionally experience depression before their menstruation (see "Premenstrual Syndrome" on pages 148–149). Often depression is experienced in recurring waves. If a period of depression lasts for more than two weeks, it would be wise to seek professional help. The causes of depression can be related to both emotional reactions to circumstances that have occurred beyond the person's control, such as the loss of a loved one through death or divorce or the loss of a job, or a chemical imbalance in the brain (known as endogenous depression). Depression may also occur when a person feels isolated from loved ones. Other causes include continuously high levels of stress, the onset of illness and the overuse of alcohol and drugs.

Symptoms

Symptoms of depression vary from person to person, but generally involve the affected persons becoming distant from the world and not wishing to take part in their usual activities. A profound sense of worthlessness in themselves and in what they do is often present, which leads to a loss of interest in everyday activities. An inability to work at their former capacity often occurs, as well as an inability to focus or do simple tasks. Episodes of depression sometimes involve frequent bouts of crying as well as strong mood swings. Physical disturbances can also occur, such as headaches, insomnia, loss of appetite and libido. Depression has also been linked to the "winter blues," also known as Seasonal Affective Disorder (SAD). One theory posits that SAD occurs because the shortening of daylight hours affects a person's personal rhythm. The rhythm between waking and sleeping is particularly disrupted when the sufferer is required to wake up when it is still dark. This lack of light is cited as one of the major causes of SAD. Light activates the body's pineal gland to stop secreting a hormone called melatonin, which helps the body sleep. If there is insufficient light, the gland continues to secrete melatonin, keeping the body feeling tired. Recognizing and treating depression is of utmost importance. If unrecognized, suicidal feelings and a reliance on substance abuse may further undermine a person's self-esteem.

Ayurvedic Treatment

It has been said that an unexamined life is a life not worth living. Though a serious and debilitating condition, the underlying value of depression is that it offers space for existential enquiry, to process and reflect on the past and integrate it into the present in a way that will enrich the future. Whether the depression is reactive (due to circumstances or events) or endogenous (as a result of internal biochemistry), the best approach is to strengthen the mind. This can be done through herbs and psychotherapy. Ayurveda often employs rejuvenative herbs such as winter cherry, shatavari, holy basil, saffron and brahmi. These are often supplemented with tailored meditation practice and body therapies such as shirodhara to balance pituitary gland function. Stimulating music, colors and gems are also effective mood elevators.

Lifestyle Changes

To alleviate depression, a shift in one's whole perspective is often required. One way to train the mind to cultivate a positive and optimistic outlook is to keep a daily diary of the blessings experienced throughout the day. This shifts the focus from negativities to those everyday blessings that can be easily taken for granted. Setting small goals and achieving them helps one to gain the momentum and enthusiasm needed to move from the stagnant, introspective gear of depression. Often, depressed people are simply unimpressed with life. Inspirational reading, counseling and pursuing a hobby can help one to regain a lust for life. Rekindling simple pleasures such as painting, hiking, singing, playing an instrument, writing or bonding with friends can brighten a dull, jaded outlook on life. Exercise is particularly effective, as it triggers the release of endorphins, the natural pleasure chemicals. It is also vital that one gets sufficient sleep, food and light. Seeking out the company of inspiring people or helping those less fortunate than oneself can help to move one's focus off the negative and put things into a more positive perspective. Sufficient exposure to sunlight is essential to eliminate depression induced by SAD. Substances that can aggravate depression include caffeine, alcohol, sugar, marijuana and nicotine.

Case Study

Evan was a 40-year-old who had suffered depression for sporadic periods throughout his life. His tendency to feel an underlying pessimism about life was further reinforced by recent job retrenchment. Evan was given a series of energizing yoga exercises called the Five Tibetans, and asked to walk in nature for 30 minutes daily while listening to a compilation tape of his favorite music. To support his adrenal and brain function, he was given an herbal jam called ashwagandadi lehyam and a series of shirodhara treatments. Psychotherapy sessions gave Evan a renewed sense of his career options, which led him to pursue his teenage dream of joining a jazz band. On the rare occasions when the blues progressed to the black cloud of depression, Evan found group meditation sessions lifted him out of his slump.

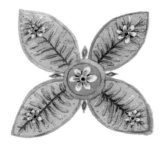

DIARRHEA

Diarrhea is the recurring elimination of overly watery stools. In Ayurveda, it is believed that stools should ideally be without strong smell, color or shape. Diarrhea is the result of bacteria in the food or water, very weak digestion or extreme feelings of nervousness. Bacteria occur in food that is poorly refrigerated or undercooked, or in water that comes from a polluted river or water system. Acute diarrhea lasts only from an hour to three days, while chronic diarrhea can persist intermittently for years.

Symptoms

Acute diarrhea caused by infected food or water is often accompanied by abdominal cramps and bloating. Associated with these pains is a loss of appetite and an increase in fluid consumption. Acute diarrhea does not usually induce a fever, while a prolonged bout can cause severe dehydration.

Ayurvedic Treatment

Diarrhea is the body's attempt to expel indigestible matter. Substances may be indigestible due to a weak digestive fire, or may be harmful, as in the case of food or water infected with bacteria or parasites. Ayurveda believes that "plugging up" the system can make things worse; instead, it aims to eradicate toxic matter (ama) while strengthening the digestion (agni). At the initial phase, a gentle bulking laxative such a psyllium husks may be given to promote complete expulsion of toxins. When this is achieved, antimicrobial herbs such as black walnut hulls, pomegranate rind, musta, grapefruit seed extract, kutaja and cloves may be prescribed. Then herbs to encourage the body to retain nutrients are given, such as bael fruit juice, nutmeg

and charcoal tablets. Once the diarrhea is controlled, herbs to reignite the digestive fire are given, which may include long pepper, cumin and ginger.

Lifestyle Changes

There is a saying in India: "If you want an unwanted guest to leave then don't feed them." This is also the case with diarrhea. Fasting from food is recommended as long as the person's strength remains. If weakness sets in, then stomachic and antidiarrheal foods such as rice soup with ginger powder and coriander leaves, pomegranate juice, unripe banana, grated cooked apple with nutmeg, guava, buttermilk and whey can be taken. Most serious complications from diarrhea arise due to dehydration. To prevent this, give plenty of the following electrolyte-rich formula. For every bowel movement, take 1 cup of room-temperature water with 1 teaspoon of lemon juice, $1/5$ teaspoon salt and 1 teaspoon of honey. When suffering from diarrhea, one should avoid hot-water bathing, exposure to the sun, oil massage and strenuous physical activity.

Case Study

Saffron, a 28-year-old woman, suffered from acute diarrhea after a trip to Southeast Asia. Initially, she was given haritaki fruit to flush out the liver and colon. She then took a combination tincture of black walnut hulls, cloves, grapefruit seed extract, wormwood and kutaja. Her diet was restricted to rice soup with a pinch of nutmeg, coriander leaves and salt. She also took cooked apples and chamomile tea with honey. Her diarrhea soon settled down.

DRY SKIN

Dry skin results from a loss of moisture from the skin. Also known as asteatosis or winter itch, the condition frequently occurs during winter when the heating of the home or office can cause cracked or scaly skin. Commonly experienced, particularly by the elderly, dry skin can cause the outer layers of the skin to peel or flake.

Symptoms
Usually, the skin feels rough and overly sensitive to rubbing. Scales may occur where patches of skin appear irritated and red. Often, dry skin affects the hands, arms and legs, and occasionally the cracks in the skin in areas such as cuticles can become cracked and inflamed.

Ayurvedic Treatment
Vata constitutions are particularly prone to dry skin, which gets worse in winter. Internal and external therapies are required to effect long-term improvement. A small quantity of ghee can be taken with each meal. Alternatively, ingesting the maximum dose of flaxseed oil or evening primrose oil daily improves the luster of the skin. Herbs to aid the digestion will facilitate the absorption of lubricants through the skin layers. The appropriate herb for this depends on the individual's doshic imbalance. Sufficient warm water mixed with a synergist such as herbal tea or fruit juice will also carry moisture to the deeper tissue layers.

Lifestyle Changes
Exercise can be used to produce perspiration to open the skin pores and to assist the proper circulation of skin nutrients. Dehydrating substances to be avoided include baked food, dried fruits or vegetables, puffed grains, tea, coffee, carbonated drinks, diuretics, wind, exposure to the sun, hot water, hair dryers and airplane flights. To manage the condition externally, try dry skin brushing to exfoliate dead skin cells, then apply warm oil to the whole body one hour before taking a bath. This can also protect the skin from drying chemicals, such as chlorine and fluoride, in the water. Vata should use sesame oil, while coconut oil is best suited to a pitta type. Kapha body types can use corn oil. Avoid chemical- and alcohol-based beauty products. Instead, a moisturizer of rosehip oil or hempseed oil and a cucumber/rosewater toner can help to seal the skin's moisture in. Ghee softens and moisturizes chapped lips.

Case Study
Heather had chronic dry skin. Now 34, she had a vata imbalance, which was evidenced by the presence of obstinate constipation. She was asked to follow a vata-pacifying diet that included plenty of ghee, warm liquid casseroles and at least 6 cups of herbal tea daily. Daily yoga exercise and sesame oil massage was diligently observed. She was also given 2 teaspoons of castor oil with a teaspoon of ginger juice to take before bed. After 10 days on this regime, she discontinued the castor oil and was given a series of small oil enemas for three days. Her skin started to feel smoother and more lubricated after one month.

EARACHE

Earaches often occur during a cold. Blowing the nose or coughing to clear the lungs may cause the ear to become infected (see pages 112–113), as the nose and throat are connected to the ear via the Eustachian tube. Viruses can infect the lining of the tube, causing swelling, which traps mucus behind the eardrum. The pressure on the eardrum causes the pain of an earache. Other causes of earache are the inflammation of the middle ear (a condition called otitis media), eczema in the ear (otitis externa, a form of seborrhoeic eczema), swimming in polluted waters and an excessive buildup of earwax.

Symptoms

Symptoms include a feeling of pressure and blockage in the ear. The hearing may be muffled. If there is a fever, it is possible that the person is suffering from acute otitis media (middle ear inflammation), and should seek professional help immediately. Untreated, this inflammation can cause permanent hearing loss. Feelings of dizziness and nausea are other indications of an infection in the ear.

Ayurvedic Treatment

An external earache can be eased by the use of antibacterial herbal drops. First steam the ear with hot water and a little tea tree oil. Then apply an antibiotic mix of garlic olive oil, which is made by heating a tablespoon of olive oil and then adding two crushed garlic cloves to it. After straining, put four drops in each ear, massaging the remaining oil around the outer ear. Mullein oil drops are an excellent alternative to this. Another specialty Ayurvedic treatment for chronic ear problems, such as an excessive buildup of wax in the ear, is similar to the Hopi Indians' ear candling technique. A cloth cigarette lined with ghee, turmeric and triphala is connected to the ear by a tube. This opens the eustachian tubes and dries up accumulated toxins in the ear. Seek medical assistance if symptoms persist.

Lifestyle Changes

As with all infections, the immune system must be supported with purifying herbs and foods such as echinacea, gooseberry, turmeric, golden seal, neem and garlic. However, these should be selected according to the individual's doshic imbalance. Avoid touching the ear, and try not to sleep on it. Swimming should be avoided until the infection has cleared. However, compresses of warm water and a little tea tree oil can be pressed on the ear for relief. Take off earrings, and reduce exposure to loud noises. A yogic breathing technique called bee's breath (bhramari) is excellent to strengthen the ear canals.

Case Study

Dominic was a 12-year-old boy who contracted an ear infection after swimming. With redness, pain and slight tinnitus, he was at the acute inflammatory stage. His ear was steamed with a mix of hot water, triphala and turmeric. Then a traditional Ayurvedic garlic and calamus oil called vacha lasunadi was dropped into the ears. A cotton wad soaked in warm water and dilute tea tree oil was placed in the outer ear for 10 minutes three times a day.

ECZEMA

Eczema is a condition of the skin resulting in itchy and inflamed areas. Usually, the affected areas are scaly, with the outer layer of the skin tending to flake off. As the areas are itchy, the skin can become further damaged and attract infection. Five types of eczema have been identified, the most common being contact and atopic eczema. Other types include seborrhoeic (see page 122), discoid and varicose eczema. Contact eczema develops when the skin is exposed to an irritant, such as some flowers (like primulas), chemical dust, some hairsprays, antideodorants, washing powders and metals, such as gold or nickel. Atopic eczema is often hereditary, especially if there is a particular history of allergic reactions, including asthma and hayfever. This type of eczema is common in children and can be triggered by stress or environmental factors.

Symptoms

Irritated, itchy patches of the skin are often eczema. Scratching the patches can lead to further infection, swelling and blisters. Once the blisters burst, a scab can form. As the condition persists, the skin in the area often thickens. Atopic eczema symptoms include redness where the skin has been in contact with the irritant. The symptoms usually subside after the irritant is removed. Atopic eczema is usually found on infants on their faces, scalps, necks, elbows and knees. As the child grows older, eczema may be found on the knees, elbows and wrists. In adulthood, long-term eczema manifests as raised, thickened areas.

Ayurvedic Treatment

Whether the cause is allergic, emotional, fungal, bacterial or unknown, Ayurveda's first tactic is to purify the gastrointestinal tract and the blood. This is achieved with herbs such as manjishta, neem, Indian sarsaparilla, *Cassia fistula*, cardamom, picrorrhiza, turmeric and triphala. The nervous system may need additional tonifying herbs, such as kava kava, winter cherry and brahmi. Once the internal channels are fortified, external oils are used to soothe the skin. Coconut-based oils with herbs reduce the inflammatory process, as well as easing the itching and oozing.

Lifestyle Changes

A diet rich in essential fatty acids, vitamins A, C and zinc has been shown to assist in eczema. This can be obtained by consuming flaxseed oil, seeds, yellow vegetables and nonacidic fruits. Foods that tend to aggravate eczema are dairy products, meat, sugar, acidic fruits, tomatoes, hot spices, yeast and alcohol. Since coriander leaves have natural antihistamines, adding some to vegetables is beneficial. Plenty of fluids, such as licorice tea, chlorophyll and aloe vera juice, can help flush out the toxins.

Case Study

Sasha was a 16-year-old girl who had suffered from eczema for the past 5 years. She had a combined vata/pitta constitution, and found the condition worsened under stress, with dairy foods and sugar and when she used soap. She was asked to stop using soap immediately, and instead to use a bathing powder made from the herb shirisha. Sasha then went on a one-week purification diet of suitable fruits, vegetables, juices and evening primrose oil. At the same time, she took triphala nightly and winter cherry to reduce stress. Daily sessions of yoga nidra relaxation were advised, followed by a relaxing 30-minute walk in shaded parkland.

EYE DISORDERS

A number of different eye disorders exist, ranging in seriousness from simple eyestrain to blindness caused by glaucoma. The most common and least dangerous eye disorder is eyestrain. Inadequate lighting while working or reading, flickering lights and light that produces glare and strong shadows can often cause eyestrain. Stress can also have a damaging effect on the functioning of the eyes, leading to the development of nearsightedness. Glaucoma occurs where the nerve carrying the images to the brain is damaged; it is caused by a blockage in the flow of clear liquid into and out of the eye. Other eye disorders include astigmatism, cataracts, conjunctivitis, dry eye and flashes. Astigmatism is the warping of the cornea. A small amount of astigmatism is quite common and can cause slight indications of blurry and distorted vision. Cataracts, which are the most common causes of vision impairment, are the clouding of the eyes' lenses. This condition can be caused by a number of factors including aging and injury (traumatic cataracts), such as a blow to the face or head; exposure to intense heat; or chemical burns. Conjunctivitis is a contagious condition also known as "pink eye," and occurs when viral infections or allergies irritate the blood vessels in the mucous membrane surrounding the whites of the eyes; the blood vessels enlarge, changing the eye white to red. Dry eye occurs when the eyes are unable to produce enough tears to lubricate the eye. This can sometimes occur after long bouts of crying. Occasional flashes are caused when the clear jelly that fills the eye rubs the retina. Another common type of eye disorder is pterigium or a callous on the eye. It develops on the white of the eye near or next to the cornea and appears as a yellow-white, raised area.

Symptoms

Symptoms of eye disorders include dry eye conditions, such as burning eyes, a feeling of scratchiness around the eyes and sensitivity to bright light, wind and smoke. Glaucoma symptoms include acute pain around and in the eye, headaches, as well as a blurring of vision. This condition requires immediate professional attention. Astigmatism causes blurry or distorted vision. People suffering from cataracts report hazy or cloudy vision. Conjunctivitis is indicated when pus forms in the corner of the eyes and on the eyelash roots. Other symptoms include burning sensations and occasionally red eyes. Flashes may take the form of bursts of bright light, star-like spots or lightning effects. There are usually no symptoms for the early stages of pterigium. Exposure to sea spray, toxic fumes or ultraviolet radiation can be some of the causes of this condition. The condition can also occur due to dryness of the eyes where an inadequate amount of lubrication is produced. Pterigium can become progressively worse if the condition is not treated, even affecting the vision if the affected area is allowed to deepen so that the growth affects the cornea.

Ayurvedic Treatment

Eye disorders can be due to an imbalance in vata, pitta or kapha. Vata disorders in the eye tend to lead to dryness, poor vision and degeneration, such as retinal detachment and eyestrain. Pitta imbalances cause burning, inflammation, conjunctivitis, yellow pus and redness. Kapha imbalances result in clouded vision, glaucoma, cataracts, thick pus and watery eyes. Ayurvedic eye treatment varies for each problem. One standard eye-strengthening and purifying treatment is triphala eyewash. Eyebright infusion is also an effective eyebath. Another therapy for vata and pitta is a technique called netra vasti. This is a procedure where a circular strip of raw dough is placed around the eyes of a reclining patient. The closed eyes are then filled with warm ghee or medicated oil. The eyes can be opened for a few minutes, then closed. This strengthens the nerves and tissues of the eyes, as well as enhancing intuition, relaxation and vision. It also helps to release painful memories from the brain's visual cortex. A drop of pure castor oil in the eyes is also healing for vata and pitta eye diseases. As shatavari is high in vitamin A, it can strengthen the eye's connective tissue integrity. Cooling herbs such as coriander seeds and leaves, roses, sandalwood and fennel are also applicable. Herbs that are high in bioflavonoids, such as gooseberry and bilberry, also help to strengthen the vision. More than just a cosmetic, Indian eyeliner (kajal) is made of camphor, ghee and castor oil, which improves the vision.

Lifestyle Changes

Ayurveda believes that the eyes are one of the first body parts to degenerate with age. Accordingly, protecting the eyes from chemicals, overstrain, sunlight and internal toxins is vital. This can be achieved by wearing protective sunglasses while outside, keeping a distance of at least 6 feet from the television, using a glare-reducing screen on your computer monitor to reduce eye strain, reading in good light and taking a break from focusing on one thing every 25 minutes. Yogic eye exercises are an excellent way to maintain clarity of vision. Trataka is another yogic technique involving candle gazing, which purifies the eyes and improves focus. Place a flame at eye level, about three feet away. Blurring your focus, gaze at the flame. Trying not to blink, continue to look at the flame until tears come to your eyes. This can be practiced twice daily. Heat also increases degeneration of the eye's connective tissue, so avoid hot hair dryers, hot water on the face, alcohol-based cosmetics around the eyes and heating foods. A diet rich in antioxidants, such as fresh fruit and vegetables, also maintains strong eyes.

Case Study

Irene was a 45-year-old pitta constitution suffering from nearsightedness and sporadic conjunctivitis. Since her conjunctivitis worsened with chilies, alcohol, tomatoes, vinegar and oil, these were removed from her diet. To cool her overheated body, she was asked to go on a pitta-reducing diet, swim in cool water and take aloe vera juice daily. She used a triphala and turmeric eyewash daily, and threw away old eye makeup to prevent reinfection. When she had the occasional relapse, Irene found placing cotton wool soaked in cold coriander seed infusion over her eyes gave rapid relief. This made by boiling 1 cup of water with 1 teaspoon of coriander seeds for five minutes. This is then strained and allowed to cool slightly before applying to closed eyes.

FEVER

Generally known as a symptom indicating a rise in body temperature, fevers usually suggest an infection. Where a dangerously high temperature occurs (over 41°C; 105°F), the condition is known as hyperthermia or hyperpyrexia. Heat stroke can result from high temperatures. A number of viral, contagious infections that cause heightened temperatures are caught by travelers in tropical climates, such as Dengue Fever and Yellow Fever. Rheumatic Fever, caused by streptococcal bacteria, is an inflammation of the heart, and can be one of the complications of a sore throat (see page 115).

Symptoms

Fever is often accompanied by a number of other symptoms, such as chills, shaking, headaches, muscle pain and a rise in the pulse rate. If it is a low fever, the cause may be part of the common cold (see pages 112–113). If the fever is high and persists for a few hours, immediately seek medical attention.

Ayurvedic Treatment

Fever occurs when the body needs to combust toxins. It also strikes when the body is free of toxins but is weak or overheated, as in sunstroke. In the initial phase of fever with toxins, Ayurveda promotes sweat and bowel movements to help remove heat and ama from the body. Sweating can be induced by keeping the patient warm, or with herbs such as ginger, cinnamon, catnip, chamomile, coriander, thyme, cloves and holy basil. If the patient's fever is dangerously high, then this approach may aggravate the situation, especially in pitta body types. The fever victim will instinctively desire what feels right. The next step is to cool the system with substances such as sandalwood, guduchi, feverfew, white willow bark, ginger, boneset, bitter herbs, red grapes, coriander seeds, coriander leaves, holy basil and rice soup.

Lifestyle Changes

Chronic low-grade fevers are a sign that the body is too weak to heal itself. The immune system may be oversensitive to a normal range of pathogens, lacking the inner energy reserves to accommodate them. The message is to rest, relax and rejuvenate the drained body and mind. Tonifying herbs, such as winter cherry, shatavari and echinacea, along with a light and nourishing diet, help to re-establish homoeostasis. Dry acupressure massage (marma chikitsa) or medicated oil massage can also help. Late nights, travel, strenuous exercise and exposure to heat or environmental extremes will only make things worse. Conversely, yoga nidra relaxation or very gentle yoga can trigger inner healing mechanisms.

Case Study

Fiona was a 29-year-old lifeguard who developed a fever for no apparent reason. She also suffered from peptic ulcers with reflux. Fiona took 2 weeks off beach watch duty and took an indoor post. This gave her body a chance to cool down. Heating items, such as tomatoes, salt, chilies, onion, garlic, red meat, fish, alcohol, citrus fruits and vinegar, were restricted from her diet. She also took cabbage juice, slippery elm and shatavari for her acidic digestion. A cooling, laxative juice from coriander leaves with a pinch of sandalwood powder and 20 ml of aloe vera juice stabilized her temperature within a week.

FLATULENCE

Otherwise known as intestinal gas, occasional flatulence is a natural by-product of digestion. However, digestive disorders can often result in chronic and excessive wind, which can cause discomfort. Poor eating habits, such as eating quickly, eating when unhappy or tense, and eating too much, are common causes of flatulence. When food or drink is taken too quickly or anxiously, excessive air is also swallowed along with the food, which moves through the stomach into the intestine, causing distension of the organs. Other causes of flatulence include poor digestion of certain foods, including milk, beans, dried fruit and cabbage. If the digestion is weak or is overwhelmed by a large quantity of food, the undigested portion of the food ferments in the intestines, leading to the creation of gas.

Symptoms

Discomfort is often experienced in the intestines as the air distends the organ. There also can be a feeling of heaviness after a meal, or a desire to have a short nap, indicating that the digestive system is having trouble processing the food. Sharp pains can sometimes be felt under the diaphragm, shooting up to the chest and mimicing the signs of a heart attack. In Ayurveda, it is believed that one of the symptoms of flatulence is mental confusion, which is understood as the elements of air and ether combining to disrupt the mind.

Ayurvedic Treatment

To tackle the problem of flatulence, Ayurveda has an abundance of useful household herbs. To increase digestive enzymes, herbs such as ginger, long pepper, garlic and asafetida are invaluable. Mild laxative herbs, such as triphala and castor oil, help to clear out fermenting intestinal toxins. Herbal oil enemas (vastis) are also an effective way of cleansing the colon. Specific carminative culinary herbs and spices are Ayurveda's specialty. Add the following to meals to reduce gas: asafetida, cumin, cardamom, fennel, coriander, ajwan and ginger. Charcoal and peppermint tablets give temporary relief in extreme cases.

Lifestyle Changes

Since flatulence is most commonly due to excess vata in the colon, a vata-pacifying diet and regime is often indicated. Vata increases as a result of stress, anxiety, dehydration, exhaustion, air travel, irregular meals and cold, windy weather. To reduce the impact of these influences, meals should be taken in a relaxed way with less talking and more chewing. Daily abdominal massage with warm sesame oil and exercises to strengthen and stretch the abdominal and back muscles can help. Gaseous foods or those that easily ferment should be minimized—especially at night. These include nuts, beans, soy milk, red meat, cabbage, raw vegetables, yeast, alcohol, sugar, milk and carbonated drinks.

Case Study

Mark suffered from gas ever since a bout of giardia 3 years ago. A powder mix called hinguvachadi (see asafetida home remedies on page 19) helped to reduce the gas. Mark also took a clove and wormwood tincture to eradicate any lingering intestinal bugs. A cleansing diet of vegetables, grains and digestive spices gave the digestion a chance to clear out built-up toxins. Mark then had a series of five oil enemas, then maintained his recovery with liver herbs including dandelion root tea and garlic.

HEADACHE

Headaches occur for a large range of reasons, including head and neck injury, tension in the forehead and shoulders, overexposure to the sun, allergens, air pollution or tobacco smoke, and overindulgence in food, alcohol and drugs. Headaches can also accompany premenstrual syndrome, sinusitis, allergies and the common cold.

Symptoms

Generally, headaches are symptoms of other conditions, such as a fever, eye disorders like glaucoma and digestive disorders. If the headache is throbbing, it may originate from stressful lifestyle conditions, while headaches that feel focused behind one eye are called cluster headaches. The pain of sinus headaches occurs behind both eyes. Headaches may be accompanied by feelings of nausea, a tendency toward irritability and sensitivity to light. Migraines are one of the most severe types of headache and are discussed on page 143. Brain tumors may be indicated when headaches are severe and recurrent.

Ayurvedic Treatment

Almost as many causes of headaches exist as there are people who suffer from them. Half the cure is in understanding the cause. The main elemental imbalance is indicated by the presenting symptoms. With vata headaches, the pain is sudden and fluctuating. It often moves around the head, and may be accompanied by restlessness, dry mouth, irritability and fatigue. Pitta headaches often involve a rise in temperature, redness, throbbing, sweating and a feeling of frustration. Headaches of a kapha origin commonly present with a congested feeling in the sinuses as well as a heaviness of the head, lethargy and depression. Vata headaches may be due to constipation, poor spine alignment, dehydration, muscle tension, intestinal gas, malnutrition, low blood pressure, low blood sugar or anxiety. Pitta headaches can be linked to liver or gall bladder disorders, anemia, impure blood, overexposure to the sun, heating foods and drinks or suppressed anger. Kapha headaches can sometimes be traced to overeating, excess sleeping, mucus accumulation in the stomach or sinuses, and grief. For vata headaches, herbal oil massage, nasal drops, oil enemas and consistent rehydration are key remedies. Useful herbs include dasamoola (10 roots combination); iron-rich winter cherry; castor oil as a laxative and Western nervine herbs such as vervain, valerian, skullcap, white willow bark or wood bettony. Pitta headaches can be treated with cooling herbs such as cumin, coriander, sandalwood, aloe vera, gentian, triphala and fennel, and cooling essential oils such as lavender, gardenia, jasmine and sandalwood. A specialized Ayurvedic therapy for pitta headaches consists of pouring tender coconut water or cool milk continuously over the forehead for at least 40 minutes (ksheeradhara). Since kapha types are often very congested, they respond to supervised steam inhalation, vomiting therapy and nasal irrigation combined with fasting to dry up mucus and toxins. Beneficial warming and stimulating herbs include trikatu (long pepper, pepper and ginger powder), fenugreek, garlic, golden seal or a traditional combination called sitopaladi churna powder (bamboo manna, cane sugar, long pepper, cardamom and cinnamon). If headaches are linked to eyestrain, follow the regimes advised in the eye disorders section (see pages 124–125). If there is a correlation with the menstrual cycle, see the premenstrual syndrome section at pages 148–149. To discount the musculo-skeletal structure as a cause, consult an osteopath, chiropractor, accupuncturist, or body worker of your preference.

Lifestyle Changes

Some simple preventative and management techniques can ease headaches irrespective of the cause, which is not always identifiable. As soon as you feel a headache coming on, take at least four cups of warm tea, such as valerian for vata, vervain or skullcap for pitta, and ginger for kapha. To subdue the pain, a paste of fresh ginger and ghee can be smeared on the forehead for vata or, alternatively, vata could drink a glass of warm water with a pinch of ground nutmeg. Kapha can drink a glass of water with a few slices of ginger to alleviate headache pain. Lying down in a cool, dark room and sleeping or listening to a guided relaxation tape (yoga nidra) can relieve the pain totally in some cases. The diet should be as simple as possible, avoiding fatty, oily, sugary, preserved or heavy foods, such as nuts, meat and dairy. Caffeine, alcohol, chocolate and preservatives are just a few of the hundreds of possible dietary triggers. An allergy test may help to identify specific triggers. Massage of the head, neck, shoulders and feet with warm sesame oil for vata, coconut oil for pitta and corn oil for kapha can dissipate causative tension. Simple yoga stretches and alternate nostril breathing (nadi shodhana) also help to relax tense muscles. Understanding one's emotional state preceding the headache can shed light on psychological origins of the condition. One can then address this through a preferred mind/body technique such as neurolinguistic programming, meditation or psychotherapy.

Case Study

Kathy was a 28-year-old woman with a pitta constitution. She suffered intermittent headaches since childhood. She found that they were worse when she suppressed anger and during the summer heat. Kathy was put on a pitta-pacifying diet and asked to drink at least 1 liter of cooling mint and vervain tea daily. She was also given a series of ksheeradhara treatments (cool milk on forehead), and asked to meditate daily for 15 minutes morning and evening. Daily self-massage with coconut and a little lavender oil was advised to cool and relax the body. Kathy also took a combination of aloe vera juice, neem, gentian and turmeric to purify her liver and blood. She found she could cool her anger by going for a walk in nature and listening to relaxing music.

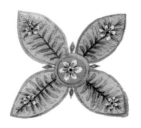

INDIGESTION

Otherwise known as dyspepsia, indigestion is a condition in which food is not fully digested by the body. Almost everyone suffers from various degrees of indigestion over a lifetime. Overeating, eating at the wrong time or in a stressed state can all contribute to indigestion. In Ayurveda, it is also believed that eating incompatible foods, such as fish and meat with milk, or beans and nuts, can cause indigestion. The first stage of digestion occurs in our mouth where, as food is chewed, it is mixed with the digestive enzymes contained in our saliva. Failure to properly chew is one of the causes of indigestion. The food then progresses to the stomach through the esophagus. In the stomach, the food is further processed with such substances as digestive enzymes and hydrochloric acid. If hydrochloric acid production is low or too high, this is another cause of indigestion. In Ayurveda, hydrochloric acid is a manifestation of the digestive fire (agni), breaking down the proteins in the food and killing bacteria. It has been observed that hydrochloric acid is produced at different rates according to the type of food in the stomach, so that the combination of foods that require different concentrations of acid, such as meat and fish with milk, should not be eaten. This is because one of the proteins will not be completely digested and will pass through to the small intestines, where nutrients from the food start being absorbed into the body. This organ is strongly affected by overeating, making it sluggish, severely slowing down digestion and impeding the utilization of nutrients from the body. The colon eliminates wastes, which, if the food was not chewed properly, are accompanied by air, causing flatulence (see page 127).

Symptoms
General symptoms of indigestion include flatulence, cramping, nausea and heartburn. Indigestion symptoms vary according to the dosha or body type involved. Vata indigestion often manifests as excessive gas, alternating diarrhea and constipation, gray toxins on the tongue, an irregular appetite and craving for stimulants such as sugar and caffeine. Pitta indigestion generally involves burning acidity or reflux in the stomach, an insatiable appetite, a tendency to diarrhea and yellow toxins on the tongue. Kapha indigestion is indicated by feelings of extreme heaviness in the stomach or esophagus, lack of appetite, fatty stools and lethargy after meals, weight gain and a whitish tongue coating.

Ayurvedic Treatment
A simple indigestion remedy for all body types is a slice of ginger, a pinch of rock salt, a pinch of long pepper (optional), and a squeeze of lime juice. Chew this mixture 5 to 10 minutes before a meal to stoke up the digestive fire for complete digestion. Vata indigestion is aided by warming carminative herbs such as asafetida, garlic, ginger, long pepper, ajwan seeds, cinnamon, nutmeg and bay leaves. Pitta indigestion requires cooling carminatives and bitter tonics such as coriander, cumin, fennel, peppermint, musta, licorice, gentian, brahmi, shatavari, arrowroot, gooseberry, and slippery elm. Kapha indigestion benefits from stimulating and warming herbs including ginger, garlic, pepper, long pepper, Indian myrrh, turmeric, cayenne, paprika, green chilies, mustard seeds, and fenugreek.

Lifestyle Changes

Ayurveda expands on the saying "we are what we eat" by adding that we are also when, why, where and how we eat. Though indigestion is sometimes due to hereditary organ weaknesses, it is more often self-inflicted and perpetuated by poor eating habits. To optimize digestion, try the following tips. Have meals at around the same time daily, but eat only if you are hungry. Avoid eating at least two hours prior to sleep and an hour prior to exercise. Minimize talking and engaging in emotional discussions during meals. Don't drink cold water directly before, with or after meals. Chew each mouthful at least 15 times. Sip warm ginger tea with each meal. Eat according to your body type, while observing the way you feel after various foods. Try to make meals from fresh food rather than just using leftovers. Avoid eating out more than three times a week. If you are overeating, think about what you are really hungry for. If you are undereating, try to inject some variety and tantalizing flavors into your diet. Enjoy a warm peppermint, fennel or cumin and coriander seed tea 30 minutes after a meal.

Case Study

Benjamin was a combination vata-pitta constitution who suffered from chronic flatulence and stomachache. At 25 years old, he had recently taken a course of antibiotics for a stomachache, but it had only grown worse. He started to improve as soon as he was put on a vata-balancing diet along with an herbal combination with asafetida, long pepper, fennel and ginger. Benjamin also started to eat with minimal conversation and in a relaxed, slow manner. He took a light protein-free dinner before 6:30 pm. Taking a room-temperature lassi (a drink made with a cup of water, $1/2$ cup yogurt and a pinch of cumin powder) after meals helped to reestablish healthy gastrointestinal flora. Before bed, Ben took 2 teaspoons of castor oil and ginger juice for 1 week to alleviate excess air and ether in the intestines. He also massaged his abdomen daily and practised yoga to release possible muscle tightness in his colon, diaphragm and stomach.

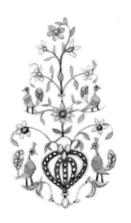

INFERTILITY

There are four major causes of infertility—inadequate sperm production, inadequate egg production, fibroids blocking the passage of the sperm toward the eggs or, rarely, the destruction of sperm by antibodies produced in either the male or female bodies. Inadequate sperm production may be caused by infection affecting the motility and number of live sperm in the semen. High temperatures experienced by the testes, especially if the man tends to wear tight, synthetic underwear, also lower sperm count. Male infertility can be further caused by a number of other factors, such as an abnormal erection; poor sperm motility or quality; a deficiency of vitamins A, B-complex, E, zinc, magnesium, protein, fatty acids, amino acids and an accumulation of toxins, such as cadmium from cigarettes; or high cholesterol blocking the penis's arteries, impeding erection. Inadequate egg production may occur if the woman is suffering from pelvic congestion, poor quality of ovum (especially if she is over 45 years of age), stress, fears, cysts, endometriosis and fibroids, the after-effects of contraception, sexually transmitted diseases (STDs) and weight problems. A study spanning from 1987-1998 showed that women who were underweight or overweight had a 60 percent decreased chance of conception, even on IVF programs. Other causes of infertility include hormonal imbalances. Inadequate levels of the hormones called gonadotrophins lower the production of eggs.

Symptoms

The most obvious symptom of infertility is childlessness. However, infertility is an issue only if a couple has been having intercourse for more than a year. Infertility is often the symptom of other conditions, such as endometriosis in the woman, which causes severe menstruation pain and infertility. For fibroid symptoms, see page 117. No indication of a slight rise of temperature during the second half of the menstrual cycle is a sign that an egg has not been made (i.e., ovulation has not occurred).

Ayurvedic Treatment

Vajikarana is the branch of Ayurveda dedicated to helping couples conceive healthy babies. Since reproductive fluids—the sperm and ovum—are considered the height of all metabolic processes, infertility is an indication of problems in other areas of the body. Tests for male infertility are less invasive and more conclusive than for females, so it is wise to check the man first. Herbs for male potency include gotu kola, saw palmetto, damiana, sarsaparilla, oats, ginseng, urad dal, licorice, kushta, garlic, gooseberry, bala, long pepper, lotus seeds, ghee, milk, almond milk, onion, palm sugar, gokshura and cloves. Natural fertility tonics for women are chaste tree, false unicorn root, dong quai, squaw vine, ginger, blue cohosh, wild yam, black sesame seeds, aloe vera, black haw, cumin seeds, dill seeds, nettle, saffron, shatavari, fennel, urad dal, and wild yam. With stubborn infertility, an Ayurvedic practitioner would suggest the couple undergo a series of purification treatments known as panchakarma (see pages 78–79).

Lifestyle Changes

You don't need to know the cause of infertility to optimize nutrition, reduce stress, take herbal fertility tonics and regain hormonal harmony. Both women and men need to regulate their natural biorhythms to ensure that all elements are in sync with their hormonal cycles. This can be done by sleeping with the moonlight shining in the room; eating according to the body's requirements, with plenty of fresh fruit, vegetables, seeds and grains; taking time for self-nurturing through yoga and self-massage and avoiding any drugs or foods that may decrease fertility. Massaging the penis and the area between the scrotum and anus (the perineum) with warm sesame oil can help to unblock tubes and bring nutrition to the area. Women can observe the guidance given for menstrual discomfort to regulate the menses. Try to see the time for conception as a sacred moment for a new soul to enter the world. A natural fertility management practitioner can help you to determine your peak fertility times, and an astrologer can assess the most auspicious time for union. The man can abstain from ejaculation for a month before conception to strengthen sperm count. On the day of conception, light, nourishing and cooling foods should be taken. The Ayurvedic text *Charaka Samhita* says the best position for conception is for the woman to lie on her back with the man on top, the woman wrapping her legs around the man.

Case Study

Jane and Dillon had unsuccessfully tried to conceive for 2 years. They were very busy and active people. Tests showed that Dillon's sperm count was fine, but he had low motility. He was advised to wear boxer shorts and to reduce his rigorous exercise routine and to stop riding a motorbike as it was overheating him and depleting his vitality. Dillon was also put on a zinc, B-complex and vitamin A supplement along with an herbal fertility jam called ashwagandadhi lehyam. Jane received counseling to discuss her fear of having a child. She doubted her ability to sacrifice her time and ambitions for a child. After some discussion, she realized that the birth of a child didn't mean death to her career. She was also given Bach flowers and regular massage to reduce her stress levels. After 4 months on a rejuvenating diet and herbs, Jane and Dillon conceived while on an island holiday.

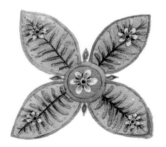

INSOMNIA

Each person has his or her own requirements of how much sleep they need to arise refreshed in the morning. Ayurveda teaches that getting the proper amount of sleep nourishes the body and promotes mental relaxation. How much sleep a person should have varies according to body type, with kapha types requiring the least number of hours of sleep. Kapha types rarely suffer from insomnia, unless they are experiencing stressful circumstances in their lives. Vata types have the most difficulties falling and staying asleep. Their ability to fall asleep is erratic, and they are easily disturbed by outside noises. Pitta types generally sleep lightly, but are generally able to go back to sleep if awoken, unless they are suffering from unresolved feelings of frustration and anger.

Symptoms

Problems falling or staying asleep or waking too early are characteristics of insomnia. This condition is often caused by a number of factors, such as premenstrual pain (see page 148) and anxiety. Chronic insomnia develops where a person is recurrently having sleep problems. Symptoms of chronic insomnia include headaches (see pages 128–129), tiredness, irritability and an inability to concentrate. Insomnia can also be symptomatic of other conditions, such as depression (see pages 118–119).

Ayurvedic Treatment

Sleep is a sanctuary where the mind and body can regenerate after the wear and tear of the day. Sleeplessness or poor quality sleep affects every aspect of one's life. Generally a result of vata or pitta imbalance, long-term sleep deprivation leads to body ache, premature aging, emotional instability, memory loss, fatigue, poor coordination, confusion, and apathy. Sleep-deprived people are a danger to themselves and others, especially in situations such as driving and operating machinery. Ayurveda uses general nervous system tonics to ground and relax vata-type insomniacs. Useful herbs include nutmeg with warm milk, winter cherry, valerian root, hops, skullcap, passionflower, kava kava, holy basil, Indian myrrh, lady's slipper and Indian frankincense. Pitta-type insomnia, which indicates more body heat and mental agitation, is treated with cooling nervines such as chamomile, gotu kola, sandalwood, hypericum, vervain and poppy seeds. Ayurvedic body therapies for insomnia include shirodhara with buffalo's milk plus gooseberry, and a crown chakra bath called shirovasti (see body therapies on page 94).

Lifestyle Changes

Common stimulants that may disturb sleep are to be avoided. These include caffeine; sugar; nicotine; chocolate; caffeinated drinks; salt; amphetamine drugs; alcohol and high tyramine foods such as smoked meats, chocolate, spinach, eggplant, wine and cheese. Foods high in tryptophan help to produce serotonin, which induces sleep. Vitamin B and C are essential for this conversion from tryptophan to serotonin. Foods containing tryptophan include milk, potatoes with skin, sunflower seeds, tomatoes, roasted pumpkin and turnips. Deficiencies in manganese, magnesium, potassium, calcium, zinc and iron can cause restlessness. Ayurveda uses specially prepared minerals called bhasmas to restore these. Try to wind down in the evening by engaging in a relaxing hobby rather than working, discussing heavy topics or doing strenuous exercise. Exercise during the day, however, can promote the body's willingness to rest. Indigestion-related insomnia will be minimized if a light dinner is taken at least two hours before bed. Applying brahmi oil on the head and warm sesame oil on the feet can sedate the nervous system. Also try a warm bath with sedative essential oils suited to your dosha, such as lavender, chamomile, ylang ylang, clary sage, frankincense, rose attar or vetivert. Daily meditation or yogic brahmari breathing before bed can help to quiet an overactive mind, often an underlying cause of insomnia. If you can't sleep, it is still important to rest the body by doing a guided relaxation or listening to soothing music. Try to make the bedroom quiet, dark and comfortable, with the head of the bed facing any direction except north and away from power points. Make realistic expectations of the day, otherwise you can feel restless due to feeling you haven't completed tasks. Visiting a sleep lab for an assessment can sometimes accurately pinpoint the problem.

Case Study

Stephan was a 30-year-old vata constitution who had suffered from insomnia since he was 16. His constant fatigue and apathetic attitude turned simple tasks into a huge effort. Stephan revealed that he was extremely stressed since breaking up with his girlfriend as a teenager. His sleep patterns were further disturbed by years of all-night music gigs. Stephan was given a series of shirodhara treatments in which warm herbal oil was poured over his forehead. This balances the pituitary gland function, which in turn reduces stress and promotes serotonin production. He was also given a tonic of ghee and winter cherry (ashwagandha) called ashwagandadhi lehyam to fortify his adrenals and nervous system. Following a regulated regime of daily yoga, self-massage, swimming and meditation, as well as going to bed at the same time daily, helped to balance his biorhythms.

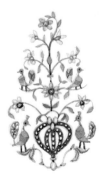

LIVER DISORDERS

The liver, the largest organ in the body, is responsible for a great number of chemical processes, such as the production of cholesterol and bile, the synthesis of protein and sugar, and the detoxification of poisons and toxins from food and environmental pollution. Liver disorders are often caused by such conditions as chronic alcoholism and excess weight. There are a number of liver disorders, including alcohol-induced liver disease, cirrhosis and hepatitis. The three types of alcohol-induced liver disease—fatty liver, alcoholic hepatitis and alcoholic cirrhosis—are caused by the excessive consumption of alcohol. Cirrhosis is caused by the replacement of healthy liver tissue with scar tissue, which inhibits the flow of blood through the organ, consequently interfering severely with the organ's functions, such as nutrient and toxin processing. Several types of hepatitis exist, including Type A and Type B. Type A is contracted through contaminated food and drink, while Type B, also known as serum hepatitis, is spread by sexual contact and using poorly sterilized needles.

Symptoms

General symptoms of liver disorders include jaundice, liver enlargement and liver failure. However, if the liver is working just slightly under par, symptoms are unobtrusive, with the condition usually indicated only by vague digestive problems and a constant feeling of tiredness. Jaundice is the yellow discoloration of the whites of the eyes, the skin and the urine. Jaundice is a disease within itself, which is due to a blockage of the bile ducts by constriction, cysts (see page 117) or stones. The reduction of bile flow, called cholestasis, is indicated by jaundice, pale stools, itchiness and easy bleeding. Fatty liver is indicated by pain below the ribs on the right-hand side. The symptoms of alcoholic hepatitis include fever and enlargement of the liver. Liver enlargement can be detected by a feeling of discomfort or fullness in the stomach. The liver rests just above the stomach. Alcoholic cirrhosis is indicated by feelings of confusion and kidney failure. Mild cirrhosis generally does not present with symptoms. However, chronic cirrhosis leads to signs of blood in phlegm coughed or vomited up, hair loss, and unintentional weight loss. Other symptoms include the development of breasts in men and ascites. Ascites is a symptom not only for chronic cirrhosis but also alcoholic and chronic hepatitis, and is indicated by shortness of breath caused by fluid retention. Liver disorders can ultimately lead to liver failure if a large part of the organ is damaged. Symptoms of liver failure include jaundice, undermined brain function, fatigue and loss of appetite.

Ayurvedic Treatment

When the liver is weak, the whole body suffers as unwanted toxins are retained and desirable nutrients are not absorbed. Though generally the bane of pitta-predominant constitutions, liver disease can strike anyone who contracts an infection such as hepatitis, or anybody who neglects diet and exercise, takes drugs or alcohol, or is exposed to environmental pollutants. Ayurveda restores liver function with a three-step approach. First, toxins must be removed from the diet and environment. The second strategy is to flush accumulated toxins from the deeper tissues. In the final phase, the liver and other digestive organs are regenerated with herbs. Prime herbs for liver problems include barberry, bhringaraja, bilberry, burdock, chelidonium, *Plumbago zeylanica*, *Phyllanthus amarus*, dandelion root, echinacea, garlic, gentian, golden seal, guduchi, punanava, picrorrhiza, red clover, St.

Mary's thistle (also known as "hairy melon"), senna, and turmeric.

Lifestyle Changes

We don't call it the liver for nothing—in order to live healthy, long lives, a strong liver is essential. Relieving the liver of its load allows it to channel more energy into removing accumulated toxins and restoring cellular function. This is best achieved by going on a fruit or vegetable fast for three to seven days. Specific foods for the liver include daikon (white radish), beets, celery, dandelion root, aloe vera, chlorophyll, bitter melon, bitter greens, ginger, globe artichoke, lecithin and ash gourd. Check your body type diet chart to figure out which ones are suitable. After the purification diet, avoid fats, oils, processed foods, refined flour, caffeine, nicotine, alcohol, drugs, sugar, salt, red meat and food that isn't organic. Avoid cooking with aluminium, amalgam fillings, exposure to chemicals and pharmaceutical drugs where possible. Essential vitamins, minerals and protein are poorly absorbed with liver dysfunction, so supplementation is often advisable. Fat-soluble vitamins B-complex, A, D, E and K, and amino acids, such as methionine, cysteine, arginine, taurine and choline, are the most common deficiencies. Avoid constipation by taking plenty of fluids and water-rich foods. Stagnation in the colon can cause extra pressure on the liver circulation, which contributes to liver pain and congestion.

Case Study

John was a 44-year-old pitta constitution with liver cirrhosis, resulting from 15 years of alcoholism. John had stopped drinking with the help of Alcoholics Anonymous, but the damage was already done. Since he had little appetite, it was easy for him to go on a vegetable juice fast for 5 days. He was also given an herbal decoction of neem, picrorrhiza, turmeric, gotu kola, brahmi, licorice, guduchi and sandalwood, along with St. Mary's thistle tablets. By strictly following the pitta-pacifying diet and regimes, as well as dealing with suppressed anger (sometimes linked to liver disorders), John was on the road to recovery.

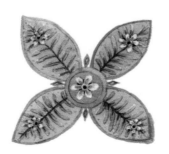

MEMORY (LOSS & IMPROVEMENT)

Memory loss can occur for a wide variety of reasons, and can range from mild short-term memory lapses to the severe and frightening memory loss experienced by sufferers of Alzheimer's disease. Otherwise known as "amnesia" and "impaired memory," memory loss can be caused by a number of factors. Common causes include aging, injury to the head, alcoholism, emotional trauma and depression (see pages 118–119). Memory, which is linked with our ability to learn, is basically our aptitude to retain and recall information. Interference in the mind's recall capacities has been linked, in women undergoing menopause, to the lowering of estrogen levels. Estrogen, one of the two female sex hormones, is responsible for language skills, balancing moods, and the ability to focus. There are two types of memory—one concerning memory for facts and dates (declarative memory), and the other relating to procedures (procedural memory), such as driving a car. One of the best ways to improve your memory is to keep your mind as active as possible—play chess or some other challenging mind game and learn new skills. Other factors that will help improve one's memory is relaxation and sleep. When people feel relaxed, they are better able to recall stored information. During sleep, the brain is processing and storing information. If this process is not completed—for instance, because the person is suffering from insomnia—then mild memory loss may be experienced.

Symptoms

Severe memory loss is generally a symptom of a number of conditions, such as Parkinson's disease, dementia, brain surgery, stroke and seizures. Memory loss is also one of the many symptoms experienced by women going through menopause. Smoking, excessive coffee consumption and drinking even small quantities of alcohol are believed to contribute to mild memory loss. Smoking also affects the memory because it decreases the levels of oxygen circulating through the brain.

Ayurvedic Treatment

Ayurveda explains that memory retention is governed by kapha, information assimilation is ruled by pitta and memory retrieval is connected with vata. Vata body types grasp concepts quickly and forget them just as rapidly; pitta is fast to comprehend and remembers well; and kapha is slow to understand though knowledge is retained for a long time. Ayurveda uses herbs, diet, meditation and body therapies to nourish and stabilize brain activity. Time-tested brain boosters include winter cherry, ginseng, cayenne, brahmi, calamus, shankapushpi, gingko biloba, holy basil, bhringaraja, gotu kola, gooseberry, milk and ghee, nasya, brahmi oil (applied to the head) and *saraswatam* powder (a combination of 10 memory-enhancing herbs.) Ayurvedic therapies to restore memory function include shirolepam, which entails applying a gooseberry paste on a shaved head for a minimum of seven days. Shirodhara, shirovasti and takradhara (buttermilk on the cranium) are also employed. (See Ayurvedic body therapies, pages 94–95.) Sometimes memory loss is due to general physical debility. In this case, full body therapies and herbs are prescribed. These help to clear mental and physical toxins and fortify neural pathways throughout the entire system.

Lifestyle Changes

A serene mind is like a still lake: drop something in and it creates a deep rippling impression. A stressed mind is like a choppy ocean, too distracted to register extra activity. We often forget vital information when under stress, as the brain is overloaded and preoccupied. Ayurveda recommends meditation or guided relaxation to still the hyperactive mind. Brain function is also impaired by poor cerebrovascular circulation. This can be improved with aerobic exercise and daily cranial massage with coconut or brahmi oil. Brain foods include tapioca, spinach, almonds, pure ghee, amino acid-rich food, and cow's milk. Toxic and oxidizing substances such as aluminium, mercury, alcohol, drugs, cigarettes, rancid fats and environmental pollutants can damage brain function and destroy brain cells. Nutrients shown to aid the memory are coenzyme Q10, essential fatty acids, vitamin B12 and iron. As the saying goes, "If you don't use it, you lose it." Hence it is essential to keep the mind's retentive power active by playing memory games, studying and focusing on absorbing present perceptions rather than dreaming about the past or future.

Case Study

A 58-year-old vata-pitta constitution, Al started to forget little things, like where he left his car keys and the names of friends. He was also experiencing stress because he was reluctantly planning to retire in the near future. Al was given brahmi and bhringaraja oil to apply to his head daily. He also took a combination of brahmi, gotu kola and gingko biloba with warm ghee and cow's milk to aid its absorption. Counseling helped Al to see the positive side to retirement as he wrote down his future aspirations including places to see, hobbies to pursue and freelance writing projects to work on. Daily qi-gong helped Al to relax and clear his mind of stressful thoughts. He also reduced his alcohol intake, which had become excessive. As a result of these adjustments, Al's memory gradually began to improve.

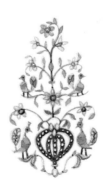

MENOPAUSE

Menopause, or "change of life," marks the end of menstruation. When a woman is in her late 30s or early 40s, the body starts gearing up for the end of the reproductive period of a woman's life. This initial stage of menopause, called "climacteric," can last for about 3 to 5 years. This phase starts the slow, gradual process of shutting down the reproductive system by starting to lower the production of the woman's sex hormones (estrogen and progesterone). By the mid-40s to early 50s, a woman will start feeling menopausal symptoms. When a woman experiences menopause varies, depending in part on her family history, when her menses started and whether she smoked. Smokers are believed to reach menopause earlier than nonsmokers.

Symptoms

The first signs of the onset of menopause are irregular menstrual cycles and heavy bleeding that occurs at unpredictable times. It is important to remember for women still in their late 30s and early 40s that menstruation may have just temporarily stopped for other reasons, such as stress, over-exercise, lack of exercise or an inadequate diet. Other symptoms of menopause may include headaches (see pages 128–129), insomnia (see pages 134–135), abdominal discomfort, backache, fatigue, memory loss, sweating and "hot flashes." Emotional disturbances are also a symptom of menopause, with some women experiencing severe mood swings, stress (see pages 152–153), irritability or depression (see pages 118–119). These symptoms may be evident for up to two years until the body is able to adjust to the loss of sex hormones. Menopause is over when a woman does not experience periods for over a year.

Ayurvedic Treatment

With a positive perspective, menopause can be welcomed as a natural metamorphosis rather than a complete imbalance of the body. While some view it as a dreaded ending, Ayurveda sees it as a "meaningful pause" before the beginning of a liberating new phase: a time when a woman's wisdom comes to fruition so she can share the wealth of her experience. Many women make a smooth transition into menopause, happy to say goodbye to the cramps, bleeding and mood fluctuations associated with the hormonal cycle. This is especially the case with healthy, fit women and those from cultures in which age is valued. Menopause can also cause fibroids to shrink and may relieve endometriosis. Endometriosis is a condition in which the lining of the uterus thickens painfully. For others, however, challenges arise at this time due to doshic imbalances. Hot flashes, tiredness, moodiness, dryness and weight gain are some common symptoms. The risk of osteoporosis, heart disease and high cholesterol also increases after menopause. If this were solely due to low estrogen, all women would experience these symptoms, but this isn't the case. Women with pre-existing doshic imbalances and an accumulation of metabolic toxins (ama) are the ones who experience menopausal difficulties. Ayurveda therefore takes an individualized approach to menopause according to the elemental imbalance responsible. Regular purification regimes (panchakarma), exercise and a whole food diet before menopause are the best safeguards against later menopausal discomfort. Herbs to balance hormones include rose flowers, shatavari, fennel, licorice, lotus seeds, cumin, wild yam, red clover, punarnava, alfalfa, flaxseed oil, dong quai and Siberian ginseng, sage and castor root. Supervised vaginal douches (uttara vasti) with oil or infusions of neem, triphala, and aloe vera can help to cleanse the uterus.

Lifestyle Changes

Effective menopause strategies depend on whether a vata, pitta or kapha imbalance exists. Vata menopausal symptoms include dryness, insomnia, osteoporosis and anxiety. Pitta problems are heavy bleeding, impatience, hot flashes and acne rosacea. Kapha symptoms may involve weight gain, water retention, depression, raised cholesterol and fatigue. These can be tackled by following the appropriate diet for the affected dosha. Following Ayurvedic daily regimes such as self-massage, yoga and meditation can help the body to maintain a natural homeostasis. Hormone replacement therapy is an option for women who are in a high-risk category for osteoporosis, heart disease and high cholesterol. Deciding upon this therapy should be an educated choice made with the awareness of possible side effects, such as breast cancer, gall bladder disease, weight gain and raised blood pressure. Natural plant hormones from herbs such as dong quai, combined with purification therapies such as herbal enemas and vaginal enemas (uttara vastis), are often sufficient to support the body through a smooth and healthy transition. Foods and supplements that can assist the process include vitamins A, B, C, E and calcium, magnesium and zinc. The mineral boron boosts estrogen levels and is present in almonds, hazelnuts, grapes, dates, peaches, honey, apples, pears and soybeans. Greens such as cabbage, brussels sprouts and broccoli are also estrogenic and antioxidant. Women with a history of breast cancer must seek the advice of a health care professional before taking high estrogen supplements, foods or herbs.

Case Study

Bernadette started to skip her periods at 53. She was a vata-pitta constitution with high blood pressure. After one year, her periods stopped completely, and she started to get hot flashes, dry skin and hair, and frequent bouts of irritability. Following a vata- and pitta-pacifying diet helped to stabilize her symptoms. She also practiced self-massage, meditation, yoga or swum daily. Bernadette thrived on a combination of licorice, shatavari, dong quai and castor roots in a ghee medium. Sage tea helped to soothe her hot flashes. She was advised to check her bone density and triglyceride levels annually.

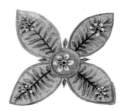

MENSTRUAL DISCOMFORT

There are two types of menstrual discomfort (or dysmenorrhea). The first type, called Primary Spasmodic Dysmenorrhea (PSD), generally occurs in teenagers and childless women. PSD is caused by a tightening of the muscle in the uterus, which constricts oxygenation and the flow of blood, leaving the uterus prone to the buildup of wastes, such as carbon dioxide and lactic acid, that increase pain. The second type is called Primary Congestive Dysmenorrhea (PCD), and is caused by toxins in the body. These toxins can occur because of food allergies (particularly to wheat or dairy products), high estrogen, and a pituitary hormone (ACTH).

Symptoms

Symptoms of Primary Spasmodic Dysmenorrhea include pain in the lower abdomen, lower backache, diarrhea, constipation, fatigue and faintness. This strong pain usually occurs during the onset of the menses. Primary Congestive Dysmenorrhea is characterized by swelling around the breasts, lower abdomen and ankles, as well as by feelings of irritability and headaches, even migraines.

Ayurvedic Treatment

Ayurveda offers some practical tips to handle the monthly menses so it doesn't cramp one's style. The average 450 periods a woman experiences in a lifetime are seen as a valuable purification of the blood and the uterus. A healthy menstrual cycle is dependent on the proper function of the endocrine glands to stimulate hormone secretion and the liver and gastrointestinal tract to break down and eliminate them. Effective herbs for cramps include cramp bark, asafetida, wild yam, kava kava, valerian, raspberry leaf, aloe vera gel and ginger. Castor oil taken before periods can help to ease congestive pain. Heavy periods are reduced with anti-pitta liver and uterine tonics like shatavari, licorice, coriander, punarnava, musta and winter cherry.

Lifestyle Changes

Try to cultivate healthy habits throughout the month. Regular sleep, daily self-massage, regular exercise and a positive mental attitude all help. Avoid the following foods: animal fats, alcohol, eggs, sugar, salt, yellow cheese, tea, coffee, soft drinks, fried foods, chocolate, cold foods and drinks, and recreational drugs. Helpful foods include monounsaturated cold-pressed oils, seeds, fresh fruit, vegetables, split mung dal and whole grains. Try to reduce activity and stress for the first three days of the period, enjoy a light and liquid diet, avoid strenuous exercise, abstain from sex, and use sanitary pads rather than tampons, as this facilitates a more complete flow. Baths in soothing essential oils such as chamomile, geranium, rosemary, fennel and sweet marjoram can reduce cramps. Abdominal castor oil packs on the stomach can also relieve pain. Helpful supplementation for some women includes vitamins A, C, B-complex, bioflavonoids, calcium, iron, magnesium and zinc.

Case Study

Natalie, 26 years old, experienced painful periods and constipation for the past year. Natalie's GP advised her to go on the contraceptive pill, but she was afraid of the increased long-term risk of side effects, such as breast cancer, liver tumors, skin pigmentation and weight gain. Instead, she adjusted her diet and took a tea of cramp bark, castor roots, fennel and shatavari one week before periods. Vitamin B_6, calcium, magnesium and zinc were also taken to help normalize muscle contractions.

MIGRAINES

Migraines are severe, recurring headaches that are caused either by allergens in certain foods, such as chocolate and red wine, or emotional distress, excessive exercise, overheating, low blood sugar, and high blood pressure. Women predominantly suffer migraines, particularly those with a family history. Migraines can occur during menopause, pregnancy or menstruation.

Symptoms

There are two types of migraines—the classic and the common. The classic migraine has symptoms of a severe headache along with numbness in the face, arms or legs, while the common migraine is only indicated by the headache. Another difference between the two types of migraine is that the classic migraine sufferer also experiences "auras." Auras include disturbances of the senses, such as seeing solid objects through a shimmering haze. The first sign of a migraine is the numbness, followed by a throbbing headache on one side of the head, sometimes on the same side as the numbness. The pain can last from several hours to several days, and recur up to three times a week. Migraine sufferers are often light-sensitive, and can experience nausea.

Ayurvedic Treatment

People predisposed to migraine attacks tend to be sensitive to particular stimuli. As with headaches, the key is to identify the trigger and avoid it wherever possible. Bright lights, sun, strong smells, suppressed emotions, food allergens, and chemical sensitivity are just some of the possible exacerbating factors. Premenstrual migraines, due to an increased fluid retention in the brain, are another common variety. As migraine is an extremely painful condition, Ayurveda may resort to an extreme cure called rakta-moksha or bloodletting. This relieves the pressure in the cranial blood vessels and removes impure blood from the area, particularly where pitta is aggravated. It is perfectly safe, pain-free and extremely effective when performed by a qualified Ayurvedic surgeon. To increase one's resistance to triggers and to subdue the vata and pitta root of many migraines, internal medicines are prescribed. Common ones include milk, ghee, saffron, sandalwood, valerian, urad dal, feverfew, wood bettony, and white willow bark.

Lifestyle Changes

Allergy testing can help to isolate the cause of migraines. Common allergens to be wary of include those found in chocolate, citrus, caffeine, cheese, red wine, food preservatives, MSG, peanuts, wheat, smoked meats, yeast, food colorings, benzoic acid, wine and the contraceptive pill. Since heat can often aggravate a migraine, it is best to wear sunglasses and a hat if exposed to the sun. It is better still to avoid the midday sunlight if possible. At the initial sign of a migraine, massage the head with sesame oil, retire to a quiet and dark room, and pull the earlobes down while yawning to release blood vessel pressure. Inducing vomiting with warm salty water may give instant relief. A few drops of warm ghee up the nostrils may help with vata-predominant migraines.

Case Study

Rob was sick of feeling sick. He experienced feverish migraines for 3 continuous days every month for the past 6 years. Pulse diagnosis identified problems in his liver as being the root cause. He was given liver herbs (dandelion root, punarnava and chitraka) along with panchakarma purification therapies to cleanse toxins from the liver.

OSTEOPOROSIS

Osteoporosis affects the bones, causing them to lose their peak bone mass until they become brittle. Although it affects men also, this condition usually occurs in postmenopausal women (see pages 140–141), and is believed to be linked to the lower amounts of estrogen produced in the body during this time of a woman's life. It also has a strong hereditary link. To keep bone tissue healthy, it is constantly broken down and replaced. Osteoporosis disturbs this balance between the breakdown and formation of new bone. The disease develops when the bone's ability to form new bone tissue weakens, allowing the breakdown of the bone to dominate. Preventative measures to alleviate the cause of osteoporosis include maintaining peak bone mass by implementing a regime of regular exercise and exposure to sunlight. Factors that diminish peak bone mass include pregnancy and immobility.

Symptoms

There are generally few symptoms of osteoporosis. However, if bones break while doing normal, everyday tasks or through minor injuries, it is important to check with a medical practitioner for signs of osteoporosis by having an x-ray. Other symptoms of osteoporosis include persistent backache and the development of a hump on the back (kyphosis).

Ayurvedic Treatment

From an Ayurvedic perspective, osteoporosis is a vata condition, with the bones becoming porous due to an excess of air and ether along with a decrease in earth. Though osteoporosis can occur at any age in both males and females, it is most common in vata-constitution women after menopause. Other things that increase the likelihood of osteoporosis include eating disorders, malnutrition, poor digestion, lack of exercise, alcohol, aluminum, cigarettes, carbonated drinks, high salt, protein and sugar intake, and steroid use. Prevention is better than cure in this case, as once bone degeneration has occurred, regaining it can be a slow and gradual process. In the meantime, the body is more vulnerable to fractures and joint diseases. To prevent osteoporosis, Ayurveda guides a person to keep their doshas in balance with an appropriate diet and a vata-pacifying regime. This is only really effective if commenced before the age of 30. Herbs to facilitate mineral circulation and deposition into the bones are used, such as ginger, long pepper and cinnamon, provided they are suitable for the body type. Herbs that increase estrogen are used to help postmenopausal women retain minerals, including red clover, alfalfa, parsley, sage, aniseed, fennel, sarsaparilla, licorice, false unicorn root, lady's slipper, wild yam, peony, black cohosh and passionflower. Herbs that are high in natural minerals can also help. Some of these are horsetail and cissus quadrangularis (colloquially known as "chain of bones"). Effective support in this approach is exercise, diet and oil therapies.

Lifestyle Changes

The best way to prevent osteoporosis is to do weight bearing exercise such as brisk walking, yoga, pump classes, or low-impact aerobics. The vital time to do this is before you are 30 years old, when the bone is still gaining density. Once osteoporosis has set in, exercise must be gentle at first to prevent fractures. Start with aqua-aerobics before progressing to cycling on an exercise bike, then walking. The regimes to regulate the menstrual cycle mentioned for premenstrual syndrome (see pages 148–149) should be observed, as women have a higher rate of osteoporosis when they miss periods frequently through their life. Mineral-rich foods should also be included in the diet, such as sesame seeds, figs, mustard greens, turnip, bok choy, kale, broccoli, almonds, Brazil nuts, hazelnuts, figs and prunes. As boron, a nonmetallic element, prevents calcium and magnesium loss, foods high in this element also assist in osteoporosis prevention. High boron foods include apples, grapes, pears, peaches, soybeans, molasses and honey. Fresh fruit, vegetables and beans rich in vitamins A, D, E, K and B-complex are also important for bone integrity. Vegetarians have a lower incidence of osteoporosis as meat is high in protein and acid, which promotes the excretion of calcium. Milk and dairy products may not be a reliable source of bone calcium, as the calcium, magnesium, phosphorus ratio increases serum calcium yet decreases bone calcium via a natural acid-buffering mechanism. This surprising finding emerged from wide-scale nutritional studies that found countries with the highest dairy food intake also had the highest evidence of osteoporosis.

Daily oil massage with calcium-rich sesame oil is essential to prevent or treat osteoporosis. Ayurveda has devised several strengthening herbal oils for this purpose using bala, ginger and urad dal.

Case Study
Lavinia underwent early menopause at 42 years of age. Since her bone density tests were a concern, she was considering taking hormone replacement therapy. Once started, however, this cannot be stopped, as the bone density can drastically plummet. So instead, Lavinia decided to try some estrogenic herbs such as red clover, black cohosh and sage. Her usual hectic lifestyle was modified with the addition of daily self-massage, guided relaxation and a 30-minute walk daily. Lavinia followed a diet that was high in minerals and vitamins, avoiding caffeine, sugar, salt, carbonated drinks and excess red meat. She drank plenty of herbal teas, such as licorice and sage, to keep her hormones balanced.

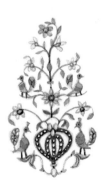

OVERWEIGHT

People are considered overweight if their weight exceeds the set standards and they do not feel fit and healthy. These set standards have been developed by various health officials to assess whether a person is overweight or obese. The term "obese" refers to weight that is over the acceptable set standard according to a person's age and height. Obesity is a condition in which there is a high level of body fat and falls within the category of "overweight." The term "overweight" encompasses both obesity and minor gains of excess weight. Excess weight can be calculated in a number of different ways, including the Body Mass Index (which is a calculation of the relationship between a person's height and weight) and the measurement of body fat. Excess weight can be caused by a great number of reasons, including overeating, lack of exercise, poor digestion caused by trauma, inattention to the body or an emotional upheaval. Genetics may play a part, as well as medical illness and medications.

Symptoms

Generally, symptoms for overweight and obese people include fatigue, little or no energy, shortness of breath, palpitations and an irregular heartbeat. Excess weight is distributed in one of two ways—across the abdomen and upper body and across the hips. This weight can come from muscle, fat or retained fluid. The most dangerous distribution of weight for health purposes is across the abdomen and upper body. One test to determine whether you are overweight is to measure your midriff. You may be overweight if your midriff measures more than 35 inches (90cm) if you are a woman or 40 inches (101.5 cm) if you are a man. Excess weight and obesity are the symptoms of a number of diseases, such as diabetes type 2 (noninsulin-dependent), heart disease, high blood pressure, stroke and problems with the gallbladder.

Ayurvedic Treatment

Ayurveda teaches that a healthy weight is achieved when a person is healthy, eschewing artificial standards to assess an ideal weight and height ratio. People with kapha constitutions will naturally be a little heavier as a result of their slower metabolisms, making them gain weight easily and lose it slowly. Weight gain may indicate water retention, hypothyroidism or ama accumulation. Whatever the cause, the focus should be on losing waste rather than weight. An ideal weight is one at which a person can access his or her optimal stamina, fitness and health. The weight of a waif-like model may be perfectly natural and effortless for a vata-type constitution, but is dangerously depleting for a kapha or pitta constitution. Carrying a bit of extra weight can promote greater longevity, providing a reserve to help counter the vata years of old age. For example, look to the gracefully aging, voluptuous Sophia Loren, a heavier kapha type. Along with diet, exercise and mental attitude, Ayurveda has some powerful fat- and toxin-reducing herbs to facilitate weight loss. These include triphala (gooseberry, bibhitaki and haritaki), Indian myrhh, vidanga, turmeric, fenugreek, ginger, asana and khadira.

Lifestyle Changes

Overeating and underexercising are the simple origins behind most weight gain. Food can be abused as a tool to push down uncomfortable emotions. Pitta body types tend to overeat to suppress feelings of stress or frustration. Vata constitutions use food as a diversion from anxiety and fear. Kapha types commonly eat for comfort or as a love substitute when lonely, depressed or bored. The best way to overcome this automatic behavior is to be conscious of the underlying emotional hunger that is being masked by physical hunger. Fostering awareness before and during eating by chewing well, breathing, remaining silent and eating away from diversions such as television helps one to focus on the body and mind's response to the process. Avoid snacking. Instead, eat a regular light breakfast, a substantial lunch and an early dinner to assist the body to digest food efficiently. Try to get variety from food, including all six tastes—sweet, sour, salty, bitter, pungent and astringent. Seek alternative sources of energy and pleasure, cultivating a taste for life rather than trying to get it solely from food. Walking on the earth, soaking up some sun, breathing in ocean air and pursuing an engrossing hobby can all help reduce a dependence on food for vitality and stimulation. A liquid juice or vegetable fast one day a week can aid the liquefaction and elimination of toxins from the system. It can also help to normalize the metabolism and appetite. A kapha diet is suitable for simple cases of weight gain. This diet suggests avoidance of animal fat, deep-fried foods, sugar, dairy, alcohol, nuts and eating out. Items that support weight loss include light, warm, bitter, pungent and astringent foods. Examples of these are apples, pears, pomegranates, cranberries, honey, beans, barley, corn, millet, buckwheat, rye, spices (except salt), asparagus, eggplant, green leafy vegetables, celery and sprouts. Drinking warm herbal teas with honey can help to cleanse the channels and allay hunger. Pranayama breathing also stimulates proper digestion, assimilation and elimination of meals.

Case Study

Dawn was a kapha body type and felt comfortable with her larger athletic build. Over the past year, however, she had gained weight, and felt sluggish and bloated. Dawn followed a kapha-reducing diet, taking triphala guggulu before bed (a combination of ginger, gooseberry, haritaki, bibhitaki and Indian myrrh). She also overcame long-term depression by joining the local water polo team and creating closer friendships. Within 2 months, Dawn was happy to reach her target weight, and felt more energetic.

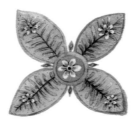

PREMENSTRUAL SYNDROME (PMS)

Premenstrual Syndrome (PMS) occurs approximately 7 to 10 days before the onset of menstruation. Some women experience PMS just after ovulation. The symptoms stop 1 or 2 days into the period. The cause of PMS is not yet known, but a number of studies are being conducted to understand this condition. Researchers are currently considering the concept that PMS is caused by changes in the sex hormones (estrogen and progesterone) levels. The changes in these levels are possibly linked to the symptoms of fluid retention in the body. Recent research by the National Institute of Mental Health (NIMH) has found that when the sex hormones were temporarily "turned off," the women in the study did not experience mood swings. A low level of certain neurotransmitters is also being considered as the cause for the emotional disturbances experienced by woman who have PMS. Other possible causes of PMS are being studied, such as psychological factors, nutritional imbalances and serotonin function. PMS can appear at any time during a woman's reproductive life, with symptoms usually occurring when the woman is in her 20s and 30s.

Symptoms

Premenstrual Syndrome exhibits both physical and emotional symptoms. Physical symptoms include fluid retention, sensitivity of the breasts, bloating, weight gain, food cravings for both salty and sweet foods, lower back pain, acne (see page 100), insomnia (see pages 134–135), headaches (see pages 128–129), migraines (see page 143) and constipation (see page 114). Emotional symptoms include irritability, feelings of impatience or being out of control, low self-esteem, depression and mood swings. The severity of the symptoms varies from woman to woman. Menstrual discomfort, dysmenorrhea (see page 142), is not one of the symptoms of PMS. The condition finally ceases upon menopause (see pages 140–141).

Ayurvedic Treatment

The cycles of the female reproductive system are a constant reminder of women's connection with the larger cycles of nature, allowing them to regularly flush out mental and physical impurities and experience richly varied moods throughout the month. Research shows that during ovulation, women are more outgoing, creative and energetic, and while menstruating, they are more introverted, hypersensitive and intuitive. It is during this transition between ovulation and menstruation that PMS tends to peak. The degree of PMS suffered depends on the level of metabolic toxins (ama), organ weaknesses and hormone imbalances in the body. The symptoms vary according to the dosha affected. Vata PMS tends to manifest as anxiety, lower back pain, insomnia, restlessness, constipation, gas with abdominal bloating and fluctuating energy. Pitta PMS may present with more anger, hunger, impatience, headaches, diarrhea, skin outbreaks and sweating. Kapha PMS often involves depression, weight gain, fluid retention, tender breasts, leucorrhoea and sluggish digestion. It is best to follow the diet for the relevant doshic imbalance along with supplementing with specific herbs. Herbs for vata PMS include nervine tonics such as winter cherry, St. John's wort, Indian myrrh and evening primrose oil. Herbs for pitta PMS are vervain, nutgrass, aloe vera, passionflower, licorice, brahmi and shatavari. Kapha PMS herbs are dandelion root, false unicorn root, dong quai and ginger.

Important nutrients that ease the symptoms of PMS include iron, protein, B vitamins (especially B_6), magnesium, chromium, calcium, zinc and magnesium.

Lifestyle Changes

Improving the quality of one's life will also improve the quality of one's periods. As explained previously, periods are interdependent on all other biological mechanisms, making them inextricably reliant on the balance of all other bodily systems. A regulated, self-nourishing routine will help to harmonize the daily rhythms of our lives, which then stabilizes the monthly menses. Healthy nutrition, sleep, exercise, rest and recreation throughout the month will significantly reduce PMS symptoms. Foods to restrict include refined flour, sugar, caffeine, chocolate, cola, fried foods, animal fats and eggs. Supportive foods are seeds, whole grains, dates, fresh vegetables and fruit, apricots, split mung bean soup, fennel, black strap molasses, licorice, cumin and chamomile tea. Self-massage helps to calm the nervous system and promotes the flow of hormones out of the body.

Essential oils that can help with PMS are chamomile, lavender, geranium, rosemary, clary sage, rose attar, sandalwood, lotus, fennel, vetivert, jasmine and ginger. Reducing work and social activities at this time relieves the body and mind of extra stress. Yoga postures for periods and guided relaxation are also highly beneficial.

Case Study

Ursula suffered from kapha-type PMS for a few days every month. She felt bloated and depressed, and she retained water. Ursula followed a kapha diet with the specific PMS restrictions. She also took an infusion of dandelion root, ginger, long pepper, pepper and cumin. A tincture of dong quai helped with the depression and B-complex with extra vitamin B_6 reduced her water retention. Baths with Epsom salts and myrrh essential oil also reduced bloating. For an energy boost, she would also occasionally take Korean ginseng. The biggest improvement seemed to take place after she started walking 30 minutes a day and reduced her work responsibilities around the time of her period.

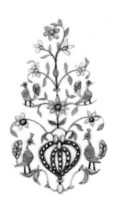

PSORIASIS

Psoriasis, a noncontagious recurrent skin disorder, is characterized by the appearance of red, scaly patches of skin. The patches usually occur on the trunk of the body and around the scalp, elbows, knees and ankles. The cause is still unknown, although the condition has been around since ancient Greek times. The word "psoriasis" is derived from the Greek word for "itch." However, it is believed that the cause could be genetic, with factors such as liver weakness aggravating the condition.

Symptoms

Red, scaly spots develop which, for some sufferers, are itchy, hot and sticky. The spots then merge into patches, and psoriasis on the scalp can be indicated by some hair loss in the immediate area and may be misdiagnosed as dandruff or eczema.

Ayurvedic Treatment

Those with a pitta constitution more commonly develop psoriasis. The disorder involves an increased production of skin cells, which relates to pitta's speedy metabolism. Though psoriasis's exact medical cause is unknown, Ayurveda links it to poor metabolic absorption of fats and proteins, which results in blood impurities struggling to escape through the skin. If the liver is strong, however, the impurities will be effectively broken down and eliminated. Therefore, Ayurvedic treatment focuses on bitter blood purifiers and liver tonics such as neem, turmeric, sarsaparilla, aloe vera, manjishta, Indian myrrh, dandelion and gotu kola. To ease the itching and remove scaliness, Ayurveda prescribes coconut-based oils with herbs such as chickweed, and cardamom. A body therapy called takra-dhara is very effective for removing heat and reducing stress. It entails the continuous pouring of herbal buttermilk over the forehead. A coconut oil with wrightia tinctoria leaves is another very effective external oil to reduce the scaliness and itch. Washing one's hair daily with chickweed shampoo is also very effective.

Lifestyle Changes

Though obstinate, psoriasis can go into remission fairly rapidly. Foods to omit include yogurt, meat, eggs, chilies, cayenne, paprika, garlic, onions, alcohol, sugar, caffeine, nicotine, refined flours, tomatoes and citrus fruits. This cools the body, reducing skin-cell hyperactivity. Daily swimming in salt water and exposing the area to UV sunlight can help. However, always wear a protective sunscreen to prevent skin cancer. Placing green clay on the affected areas for 20 minutes daily, then washing it off with cold water draws toxins from the subcutaneous layer. A diet rich in vitamin A, C, D, B-complex, essential fatty acids, calcium, magnesium and zinc is beneficial. Since stress aggravates psoriasis, cultivating stress-management techniques such as meditation, guided relaxation or tai chi is important.

Case Study

Jason was a 37-year-old pitta constitution who had suffered from psoriasis on the scalp and face since a teenager. He was given a chickweed, sandalwood and coconut-based shampoo to clear the scalp scales and itching. He applied coconut and evening primrose oil to his face. The biggest dietary change was to give up alcohol. He was happy to shave his head temporarily, and go for a daily swim in the sea. After 3 weeks of this regime, Jason's skin was clearer than it had ever been.

SINUSITIS/HAYFEVER

Sinusitis is the inflammation of the sinus passages, which are located above the eyebrows, next to the nose and near the base of the skull. Acute sinusitis is quite common, often occuring together with a cold. Chronic sinusitis, in which the symptoms are milder but the condition lasts longer, is believed to be caused by a fungal infection, according to new research. Hayfever, also known as seasonal allergic rhinitis, is an inflammation of the nasal passages, as well as other membranes in the eyes and throat. This condition is caused by an allergic reaction to airborne pollens and molds.

Symptoms

Acute sinusitis is indicated by fever, mucous congestion in the nasal passages, headaches, fatigue, sore throat (see page 112), pain behind the eyes and hypersensitivity to light. Chronic sinusitis is often a recurrent condition in which symptoms of severely blocked nasal passages, pain in the face and a sense of heaviness in the area are present. Hayfever symptoms include sneezing, stuffy nose, irritated eyes and an itchy feeling in the throat.

Ayurvedic Treatment

Sinusitis and hayfever are predominantly caused by a vata and kapha imbalance. Vata aggravation leads to hypersensitivity of the capillary membranes, with the resultant swelling and mucus resulting from accumulated kapha. Sufferers of sinusitis and hayfever have weak, overactive autoimmune systems due to toxins coating the channels. This creates a fertile field in which allergens flourish. The Ayurvedic approach is to cleanse the membranes, balance the immune response and strengthen the membranes' resistance. Cleansing is done with practices such as supervised vomiting (vamana), nasal irrigation with warm salty water (jala-neti), eye baths and eye drops. Colon cleansing is also important using herbs such as triphala, castor oil or senna. The immune response can be pacified with herbs such as coriander leaves, shirisha, turmeric, black cumin, fenugreek, holy basil, golden seal and echinacea. To fortify membranes, there are excellent Ayurvedic nasal drops called anu thailam, containing 28 herbs, goat's milk and sesame oil. Alternatively, warm ghee can be dropped in the nostrils.

Lifestyle Changes

To overcome hayfever and sinusitis, the irritant should be identified and eliminated. However, sometimes the irritant isn't obvious, or it is impossible to avoid. Some ways you can reduce common household allergens are to cover mattresses, steam clean or remove carpets, avoid using curtains, keep pets outside, do not keep fresh flowers, clean mold from the bathroom regularly and use chemical-free cleaners. Food allergies are another trigger for hayfever. Common trigger foods include nuts, dairy, shellfish, processed food, red wine and refined flours. Foods that act as natural antihistamines and channel dilators can be taken. These include onions, garlic, licorice, chili, horseradish, coriander leaf and parsley.

Case Study

Joel was a 31-year-old hayfever sufferer with a vata constitution. He was noticeably worse in spring and after consuming dairy products. He prepared the coriander chutney described in coriander home remedies (see page 31), taking it daily with lunch. Joel also practiced nasal irrigation and used anu nasal drops every morning. These strategies coupled with the elimination of dairy from his diet made a marked improvement on Joel's symptoms.

STRESS AND HYPERTENSION

Stress is a very individualised response. We experience stresses from a bewilderingly wide range of sources, from the anxieties associated with work, such as deadlines, constant performance anxiety, insufficient financial reward, and competition, to the demands placed on us by the environment, such as pollution, exposure to toxins, and chemicals in the food and air, as well as stress from relationships. Stress is divided into two types. One is called positive stress (eustress), which actually supports a person's well-being. The other type of stress is distress, which has a number of negative effects on physical and mental health. Hypertension, a condition that features high blood pressure, is caused by such reasons as excess weight (see pages 146–147), cigarette smoking and heavy consumption of alcohol. Normal blood pressure should be 130 for the top (systolic) reading and 80 for the bottom (diastolic) reading. Systolic refers to the pressure generated as the heart is beating, while diastolic indicates the pressure when the heart is at rest. If it is not treated, hypertension can lead to complications such as heart problems and strokes.

Symptoms

Stress is often a symptom of other diseases and conditions, such as heart conditions, poor digestion, headaches, lack of focus, depression, high blood pressure, high cholesterol levels, diabetes, insomnia (see pages 134–135), menstrual irregularities, premenstrual syndrome (see pages 148–149) and Chronic Fatigue Syndrome (see pages 108–109). Stress is also one of the factors of hypertension. Hypertension rarely has symptoms, and is generally discovered when the sufferer is being examined for something else. Possible symptoms include fatigue, nausea, heart palpitations, headache at the back of the head, excessive perspiration, and nose bleeds.

Ayurvedic Treatment

Faced with physical or emotional challenges, our natural instinct is to react with the flight, fight or fright response. This reaction occurs through the secretion of stress hormones, such as adrenaline, from the adrenal glands. Periods of prolonged stress can cause a syndrome called "adrenal exhaustion," a vata imbalance resulting from the excessive secretion of stress hormones. This makes us hypersensitive to stress, as we don't have the reserves to respond effectively anymore, a dilemma experienced by many sufferers of Chronic Fatigue Syndrome (see pages 108–109). Ayurveda teaches that humans are different from animals in that we can rationalize situations rather than automatically reacting at the whim of baser instincts such as fear or anger. By viewing challenges from a positive perspective rather than always feeling threatened, we can alleviate most stresses. Welcoming every challenge as an opportunity to learn and deepen one's character makes every experience enriching. This stance requires faith that in the long term, whatever happens to us is for a meaningful and beneficial purpose, allowing us to relinquish ultimate control of others or situations. Working as if everything depended on us, but feeling like everything depends on divine forces, allows a kind of active detachment that greatly relieves stress. As the saying goes, "For peace of mind, resign as the general manager of the universe." While cultivating this new perspective, Ayurveda offers herbs to manage the hypertension, nervous debility and anxiety often associated with stress. These include arjuna, snake root, chamomile, vervain, valerian, winter cherry, ginseng, hawthorn berry, brahmi, licorice and garlic. Body therapies are invaluable for managing and preventing stress and hypertension. Massage releases accumulated tension from the body, leaving one more relxed and serene. Shirodhara, shirovasti and navarakizhi are also used to balance the pureal, pituitary and adrenal glands which govern stress and blood pressure levels.

Lifestyle Changes

Ayurveda excels in teaching ways to diffuse and avoid stress. We can reduce stress by keeping daily goals realistic, managing money sensibly, looking after our health, limiting exposure to the news, avoiding negative company, and sharing burdens with a loving partner. A relaxed body is the gateway to a serene mind. Whenever stress starts to mount, take three deep breaths while mentally saying—"calm." Relax the shoulders and facial muscles while keeping a tranquil expression. This body language actually triggers the release of relaxing and pleasurable neurotransmitters throughout the body, reducing stress accumulation and making your cells smile. To make this level of relaxation readily accessible, daily self-massage, meditation, yogic breathing (pranayama), qi-gong, yoga, chanting or prayers are invaluable. Peaceful music is perfect for soothing the nervous system. Warm baths with Epsom salts and calming essential oils such as lavender or chamomile help to release physical tension. Renting a funny or sad video or reading a book can help us to have a good laugh or cry, which often releases pent-up stress. Keeping a balance between work, leisure and rest is essential. Taking time out for a holiday or a fun hobby can act as a panacea for stress and hypertension.

Case Study

George was a corporate executive with a pitta constitution. He was suffering from stress that resulted in high blood pressure, headaches and psoriasis. He also had a volatile temper that created havoc at work and home. Since George hadn't taken a holiday in 6 years, that was the first prescription. Instead of medication, he was interested in meditation, so George went to a yoga retreat in a beautiful location where he could receive lots of massage, exercise and meditation instruction. This two-week sojourn was just what George needed to change his outlook on life. He decided to reduce his working hours to spend more leisure time with his family and friends. To keep his blood pressure under control, George cut out alcohol and stimulants such as sugar, salt, caffeine and nicotine.

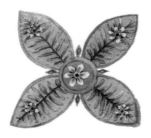

URINARY TRACT INFECTIONS

Although most urinary tract infections are not serious conditions, they cause discomfort and burning sensations during urination. Usually suffered by women, the infections are caused by bacteria, which often come from the colon and live on the skin around the rectum. Sexual intercourse and pregnancy are considered two of the causes of the bacteria spreading from the rectum to the urethra. The bacteria travels up the urethra to the bladder. Another cause of urinary tract infections is habitually resisting the urge to urinate. By doing so, the bladder gradually extends and weakens, which leads to some urine being left in the bladder. The presence of urine in the bladder after urination increases the chance of infection, as the stale urine creates a stagnant environment in the bladder.

Symptoms

Symptoms of urinary tract infection include a strong urge to urinate and a burning sensation in the urethra when urinating. Sometimes blood may be found in the urine. Pain may also be experienced, particularly in the lower abdomen, lower back and in the urethra.

Ayurvedic Treatment

Ayurveda sees urinary tract infections as a sign that the body is acidic or toxic. Bacteria or fungus proliferates in an ama-filled body, resulting in the burning, itchiness and pain of a urinary tract infection. Pitta constitutions are more predisposed to this condition with their increased tendency to acidity and inflammation. In conjunction with an alkaline diet, some powerful antibacterial herbs can help eliminate the infection. These include uva ursi, buchu, sandalwood, Indian myrrh, couchgrass, gokshura, calendula, golden seal and neem. Herbs often used to soothe and strengthen the urinary tract are cornsilk, dandelion root, marshmallow, alfalfa, horsetail, bala and shatavari. An infusion of equal parts fennel, coriander and cumin seeds can be very effective as well. Try triphala, senna or slippery elm bark powder to flush out acidic digestion.

Lifestyle Changes

Since urinary tract infections thrive in excessive heat, management involves protection from the sun, a pitta-pacifying diet and lukewarm rather than hot baths. Specific foods that can help alkalize the system include barley water, coconut water, cranberry juice, rice and almonds. Wash the area with tea tree soap or very diluted tea-tree-oil water after going to the toilet rather than using toilet paper, which can spread the infection. Condoms, sex, synthetic underwear and tampons can all aggravate urinary tract infections. A hipbath in juniper, lavender and a little tea tree essential oil can ease the burning. Supplements such as vitamin B-complex, calcium ascorbate, echinacea and zinc will assist the immune system to eliminate the infection.

Case Study

Anna had acidic reflux and a recurrent infection of the urinary tract over the past 3 months. As she was a pitta constitution, she was advised to follow the pitta-pacifying diet, particularly avoiding acidic fruits, tomatoes, chilies, red meat, alcohol and vinegar. She took triphala nightly, along with a combination of bala, shatavari and slippery elm powders three times a day. Drinking 1 liter of an infusion of corn silk, buchu, uva ursi and barley water for a week also helped her infection and reflux to clear.

WORMS

Worms usually enter the body through food, water or contact with an infected person or animal. Hookworms, which have hook-like teeth, live in the small intestines, feeding on the blood and producing eggs that are usually defecated out of the body. Threadworms, which look like tiny bits of thread, are another common type of infestation. Tapeworms are long and flat and can cause cysts in a number of areas of the body, such as the lungs and the liver. Roundworms are one of the largest parasites, resembling earthworms.

Symptoms

General symptoms for worms include dark circles around the eyes, grinding of the teeth at night and excess salivation. Usually, there are no symptoms for hookworms. They may be indicated by the presence of diarrhea and fatigue. An advanced case of hookworms can cause anemia, which is seen by the unusually pale skin. Threadworms cause intense itching around the anus, particularly at night, which can lead to sleeplessness. People with tapeworms generally do not have any symptoms; however, hunger, abdominal tenderness, diarrhea and anemia can indicate the presence of this parasite. Roundworms can stay in children's systems for years, causing possible malnutrition. For all parasite infestations, the stools usually exhibit signs of the parasite's eggs.

Ayurvedic Treatment

Since worms are a common occurrence in India, Ayurveda has developed very potent remedies to treat these irritating infestations. The herbal remedies are all bitter blood purifiers, which are sometimes difficult to feed to children, though the powder can be placed in capsules. Another alternative to herbs is homoeopathic Cina, which is usually very effective. Herbs administered for worms include garlic, neem, vidanga, onions, grapefruit seed extract, black walnut hulls, wormwood, pomegranate bark and cloves. When worms have settled in the liver, then liver herbs such as picrorrhiza, gentian and turmeric are used. To completely cleanse the body of worms, a laxative, such as triphala or castor oil, should be taken for a minimum of three consecutive days.

Lifestyle Changes

Sweet and sour foods create a sticky internal environment in which worms love to settle. To get rid of the worms, reduce sweet and sour foods, such as sugar, refined carbohydrates and citrus fruits, and replace them with plenty of green leafy vegetables and seeds. Pomegranate juice offers excellent protection against all worms. Grated carrot is effective against threadworms, and papaya seeds or the sap from the unripe fruit is used to treat roundworms. Sesame seeds and pumpkin seeds are specific medicine for tapeworms. Avoid the common sources of infection, such as animals, meat, seafood and dirt. Adopt a vegetarian diet (especially when traveling), and wear shoes and gloves when in the garden. As worms can cause malnutrition, all major vitamins and minerals, along with acidophilus powder, should be supplemented until digestive strength is regained.

Case Study

Gopal was a 6-year-old boy who loved to play trucks in the sandpit; unfortunately so did the hookworms! He was given 3 neem leaves a day along with capsules with vidanga and cloves in them. After 2 weeks on this treatment, he was given a small dose of triphala to flush the worms out.

Glossary

agni—a Sanskrit term for fire. In Ayurvedic medicine, it refers to the metabolic and digestive fire concentrated in the stomach, which is essential to the well-being of the body.

agasthya rasayana—an ancient rejuvenation jam.

ajwan—a Sanskrit term for wild celery seeds that are most useful as a digestive aid.

ama—a Sanskrit term for toxins often caused by poor digestive fire and emotional imbalances.

antispasmodics—herbs, such as asafetida, that relieve spasms, for example in the bronchial tubes and uterine muscles.

anupana—the adjunct given with an herb to determine it effectiveness for a particular condition.

anu thailam—Ayurvedic nasal drops.

aphrodisiacs (vajikarana)—substances such as urad dal that rejuvenate the sexual organs.

asana—a term referring to yoga postures.

ashwagandadhi lehyam—a fortifying jam containing winter cherry.

astringents—herbs, such as turmeric, that have a drying effect on the body, especially helpful in stemming the flow of blood from a wound or stopping diarrhea.

bael—a fruit, known in Sanskrit as bilwa, which is used to alleviate digestive disorders.

bala—the Sanskrit term for Indian country mallow, which is used as a tonic and a rejuvenative for vata disorders, such as nervous system conditions.

bamboo manna—known in Sanskrit as vamsha rochana, a milky substance from the bark of the bamboo plant. It is useful for healing lung disorders.

bhasmas—Ayurvedic tinctures made from gems that have been burnt into ash.

bhringaraja—the Sanskrit term for a herb known for its excellent properties for the hair.

bibhitaki—a rejuvenative herb, also known as Beleric Myrobalan, which helps alleviate mucus congestions.

Cassia fistula—a type of senna.

chakras—energy centers that run through the middle of the body, from the base of the spine to the top of the head.

chelidonium—a Western liver herb.

chitraka—a Sanskrit term for the root and seeds of *Plumbago zeylanica* used to alleviate gas, rheumatism, colitis and joint pains.

churna—a Sanskrit word for Ayurvedic herbal powders. These powders are useful in the preparation of certain Ayurvedic combinations that require a number of different herbs, such as triphala (see page 159).

chyavanaprasham—a Sanskrit term for one of the best rejuvenating jams in Ayurvedic medicine, containing gooseberry and ghee.

Cissus quadrangularis—a tendril climber plant also known as "bone setter."

dasamoola—a combination of ten roots given to debilitated patients.

decoction (kashayam)—a method of preparing herbs, which involves boiling them for hours until the liquid is reduced to a quarter of its original amount.

diuretics—herbs, such as *Tribulus terrestris*, that are useful to remove excess fluids from the body by increasing urination.

doshas—a Sanskrit term for the three major constitutions—vata, pitta and kapha. Each dosha has its own physical, emotional and intellectual characteristics. The three doshas are collectively called tridoshas (see tridoshic below).

emollients—herbs, such as marshmallow, that soothe the skin.

Epsom salts—otherwise known as hydrated magnesium sulphate, are often used in baths for drawing out toxins through the skin.

ether—one of the five elements that make up the world according to Ayurvedic principles. Ether is basically the space between matter, from the space between the atoms to the space between planets.

euphorbia hirta—a plant, also known as Queensland asthma weed, which is an effective bronchodilator for respiratory conditions.

expectorants (kasa-svasahara)—herbs, such as licorice, that help the body to expel mucus from the nasal passages, throat and lungs.

extract—a method of preparing herbs by using solvents or evaporation to extract the healing qualities of the herb from the leaves, roots or stems of the herb.

false unicorn root—a tonic that helps regulate menstruation and alleviate female reproductive disorders.

ghee—clarified butter, which is prepared from unsalted butter. Ghee is believed to be of enormous therapeutic benefit, able to enhance ojas (see page 158).

ghrithams—a Sanskrit term referring to herbal ghee preparations.

gokshura—a Sanskrit term for an oriental herb useful for urinary tract infections. It is also known in Latin as *Tribulus terrestris*.

gotu kola—a herb, also known in Latin as *Centella asiatica*, that has similar properties to Bacopa Monniera (Brahmi).

guduchi—a plant, whose roots and stems are used to treat immune diseases.

gulikas—a Sanskrit term referring to Ayurvedic herbal tablets.

Gymnema sylvestre—a Latin name for a plant, whose roots and leaves are used for aiding in the treatment of diabetes. Known as sarpa-darushtrika in Sanskrit.

haritaki—an important Ayurvedic herb for improving the mind, stabilizing the nerves and aiding digestion.

Infusion (hot—phanta; cold—sheeta kashaya)—a hot infusion is a method of heating herbs in water over a low flame until the water reaches boiling point; a cold infusion is a method of steeping the herbs in cold water for over an hour.

kapha—a Sanskrit term referring to one of the three doshas, which is a combination of the elements of water and earth.

kashaya/kashayams—a Sanskrit term referring to Ayurvedic decoctions (see above).

khadira—an astringent herb with the Latin name *Acacia catechu*.

kushmanda rasayana—a rejuvenative jam for the respiratory system.

kushta—a Sanskrit term for Costus, the root of which is used for the treatment of asthma, skin diseases and rheumatism.

kutaja—a Sanskrit term for a herb that is given for diarrhea and parasites. Its Latin name is *Holorrhena antidysenterica*.

laxatives—herbs, such as fennel seeds, that encourage the bowels to move, which is useful in such conditions as constipation.

mahanarayana—an Ayurvedic herbal oil combination.

manjishta—the Sanskrit term for Indian madder, the root of which is used to purify the blood.

musta—a Sanskrit term for a plant also known as nutgrass, which is used to alleviate menstrual pain and stimulate liver function.

nasya—a Sanskrit term referring to the Ayurvedic practice of taking certain medicine through the nose.

nervines—herbs, such as valerian, that either stimulate or calm the nervous system.

neuralgia—the pain associated with a nerve that has been pinched or irritated.

ojas—a Sanskrit term for the subtle essence that results from the creation of seven types of body tissues, and is the source of the body's immunity and fertility.

palm sugar—unrefined sugar extracted from palm tree trunks.

panchakarma—a Sanskrit word referring to a series of five powerful Ayurvedic treatments to purify the body. Some of its treatments include nasya (see above), oil enemas and supervised vomiting.

phanta—a Sanskrit term referring to hot infusions (see also **infusion**).

picrorrhiza—a shortened Latin term (*Picrorrhiza kurroa* benth) for a herb known in Sanskrit as katuki which is used to treat liver disorders, skin diseases and constipation.

pitta—a Sanskrit term referring to one of the three doshas, which is a combination of the elements of fire and water.

prakriti (or prakruti)—Sanskrit terms that can be used interchangeably to refer to the inherent nature of an individual's dosha or the general nature of the universe.

punarnavadi (or punarnava)—a cooling, diuretic herb, also know in Latin as *Boerhavia diffusa*, which is an excellent liver tonic.

purgatives—strong laxative herbs, such as castor oil, which are taken orally to help move the bowels.

rasayana—a Sanskrit term referring to a series of rejuvenating treatments to promote longevity and rejuvenate the body.

rasnadi—an expectorant herbal powder used externally or inhaled for respiratory conditions.

rock sugar—an unrefined form of sugar which is also known as rock candy.

sama—a Sanskrit term for ama.

Sanskrit—the ancient literary language of India.

saptasaram—a combination of seven herbs used to restore the flow of air and ether in the body's channels.

saraswatam—a herbal combination to stimulate cerebro vascular circulation and to restore mental functions.

shankhpushpi—a plant, known in Latin as *Clitoria ternatea*, which is used in the treatment of reproductive imbalances, epilepsy, memory problems and nervous disorders.

sheeta kashaya—a Sanskrit word referring to cold infusions (see also **infusion**).

sheetali—a cooling yogic breathe that involves inhaling through a cooled tongue

shirisha—an astringent herb, known in Latin as *Albizzia lebbek*, which is used for diarrhea and allergic reactions.

Shiva—supreme yogi

sitopaladi churna—one of the traditional Ayurvedic herbal powders used for treatment of colds and flus.

Solanum xanthocarpum—a Latin term for a herb, known in Sanskrit as kantakari, which is used to treat asthma, kidney problems and constipation.

soma—a Sanskrit term that corresponds with the element of water and governs the nerves and mind.

squaw vine—a reproductive tonic herb used extensively by the American Indians.

stimulants—herbs, such as ginger and pepper, which improve circulation and strengthen the metabolism.

svarasa—a Sanskrit term referring to a method of preparing herbs as a fresh juice.

thailam—a Sanskrit term for Ayurvedic herbal oils.

toners—herbs, such as aloe vera, that help to tighten and revitalize the skin.

tonics (rejuvenative—rasayana karma)—herbs, such as winter cherry, that aid the general condition of the body by renewing the body and mind.

tridoshic—a Sanskrit term that refers to herbs, foods, attitudes and mental states that are beneficial for all doshas.

trikatu—a Sanskrit term referring to a combination of long pepper, black pepper and dried ginger.

triphala—a Sanskrit term referring to a combination of gooseberry, bibhitaki and haritaki.

urad dal—a high protein legume.

vasa—a plant, also known as Malabar Nut and in Latin as *Adhatoda vasica*, which is useful for respiratory and circulatory conditions.

vata—a Sanskrit term referring to one of the three doshas, which is a combination of the elements of air and ether.

vati—a Sanskrit term referring to Ayurvedic herbal tablets.

vidanga—a herb used for the elimination of parasites as well as the treatment of indigestion.

Vishnu (Lord)—the Hindu God responsible for sustaining the universe. Lord Dhanvantari, the Celestial Physician who is the divine origin of Ayurveda, is believed to be a reincarnation of Lord Vishnu.

Botanical Index